D1475457

Refractive Cataract Surgery and Multifocal IOLs

Edited by
R. Bruce Wallace III, MD

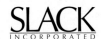

6900 Grove Road • Thorofare, NJ 08086
an innovative information, education, and management company

Publisher: John H. Bond
Editorial Director: Amy E. Drummond
Editorial Assistant: William J. Green

The procedures and practices described in this book should be implemented in a manner consistent with the professional standards set for the circumstances that apply in each specific situation. Every effort has been made to confirm the accuracy of the information presented and to correctly relate generally accepted practices. The author, editor, and publisher cannot accept responsibility for errors or exclusions or for the outcome of the application of the material presented herein. There is no expressed or implied warranty of this book or information imparted by it.

Care has been taken to ensure that drug selection and dosages are in accordance with currently accepted/recommended practice. Due to continuing research, changes in government policy and regulations, and various effects of drug reactions and interactions, it is recommended that the reader review all materials and literature provided for each drug, especially those that are new or not frequently used.

Any review or mention of specific companies or products is not intended as an endorsement by the author or the publisher.

Refractive cataract surgery and multifocal IOLs / [edited by] R. Bruce Wallace III
    p. ; cm.
    Includes bibliographical references and index.
    ISBN 1-55642-460-4 (alk. paper)
    1. Cataract--surgery. 2. Intraocular lenses. 3. Eye--Refractive errors--Surgery. I.
Wallace, R. Bruce
    [DNLM: 1. Cataract Extraction--methods. 2. Lens Implantation, Intraocular. 3. Lenses,
Intraocular. 4. Refractive Errors--surgery. WW 260 R3317 2001]
    RE451 .R437 2001
    617.7'42059--dc21
Printed in Canada
Published by: SLACK Incorporated
                     6900 Grove Road
                     Thorofare, NJ 08086 USA
                     Telephone: 856-848-1000
                     Fax: 856-853-5991
                     www.slackbooks.com

Last digit is print number: 10   9   8   7   6   5   4   3   2   1

DEDICATION

This book is dedicated to my wife, Pam. Thank you for your love and friendship and for sharing "our time" with the writing of this book.

Bruce

CONTENTS

ACKNOWLEDGMENTS

Refractive Cataract Surgery and Multifocal IOLs has been a collaborative effort, made possible by knowledgeable coauthors and their dedicated staff members. Their willingness, even eagerness, to share their experiences and advice has been a true inspiration.

I am deeply indebted to SLACK Incorporated, especially Viktoria Kristiansson, John Bond, and Peter Slack, for their support and encouragement. I especially want to thank two of my devoted staff members for the tireless energy they expended on this project, Debra Moore and Anna Johnson.

Our principle motivation to publish this book has come from experiencing the joy of happy postoperative patients. I am grateful to have a superlative refractive cataract surgery team at Wallace Eye Surgery, headed up by Dr. Robert Crotty and Marcia Hesni.

ABOUT THE EDITOR

R. Bruce Wallace, III, MD is medical director of Wallace Eye Surgery in Alexandria, Louisiana. He is an assistant clinical professor of ophthalmology at Tulane School of Medicine in New Orleans.

Dr. Wallace has been a principal investigator for a variety of intraocular lenses including multifocal IOLs manufactured by Alcon, Allergan, 3M, and Pharmacia. He continues to be an advisor to ophthalmic companies for IOL design, phacoemulsification equipment, and other surgical instrumentation. Starting in 1990, Dr. Wallace was editor of Target: Emmetropia in *Ocular Surgery News*, one of the first series of articles devoted to refractive cataract surgery. He has authored numerous journal articles and book chapters and has lectured extensively on methods to enhance phacorefractive procedures.

Dr. Wallace is past president of the American College of Eye Surgeons and the Society for Excellence in Eyecare and serves on the editorial boards of *Ocular Surgery News*, *Ophthalmology Management*, *Review of Ophthalmology* and the *Video Journal of Ophthalmology*.

Dr. Wallace and his wife, Pam, have two sons, Bill and Jim.

Contributing Authors

William P. Burnham, OD
Zeiss Humphrey Systems
Dublin, California

Kurt A. Buzard, MD
Assistant Clinical Professor of
Ophthalmology
University of Nevada–Las Vegas
Las Vegas, Nevada

David F. Chang, MD
Clinical Professor of Ophthalmology
University of California–San Francisco
Los Altos, California

Tom M. Coffman
Private Practice
Lake Worth, Florida

David M. Dillman, MD
Private Practice
Danville, Illinois

Philippe Dublineau, MD
Angers, France

I. Howard Fine, MD
Associate Clinical Professor of
Ophthalmology
Oregon Health Sciences University
Eugene, Oregon

William J. Fishkind, MD
Clinical Professor of Ophthalmology
University of Utah
Tuscon, Arizona

Kenneth J. Hoffer, MD
Clinical Professor of Ophthalmology
UCLA Jules Stein
Santa Monica, California

Cynthia J. Kendall, BMET, RDMS,
ROUB
Innovative Imaging
Sacramento, California

William F. Maloney
Associate Clinical Professor of
Ophthalmology
University of California–Irvine
Vista, California

Ivan Marais, MD
Senior Consultant
Johannesburg Hospital
Johannesburg, South Africa

Louis D. Nichamin, MD
Private Practice
Brookville, Pennsylvania

Randall J. Olson, MD
Assistant Clinical Professor of
Ophthalmology
University of Utah
Salt Lake City, Utah

Robert H. Osher, MD
Cincinnati Eye Institute
Cincinnati, Ohio

Kevin L. Waltz, MD
Assistant Clinical Professor of
Ophthalmology
Indiana University
Indianapolis, Indiana

Preface

No banner headlines in *Ocular Surgery News* announced "The First Refractive Cataract Surgery Has Been Performed!" Instead, we have been experiencing this historic evolution almost imperceptibly. Newer methods in cataract surgery have acted like building blocks toward the acceptance of refractive cataract surgery. Sir Harold Ridley's first IOL was a giant step forward, yet it took other technologies to allow IOLs to finally take their rightful place in visual rehabilitation. With surgical microscopes, phacoemulsification, viscoelastics, circular tear capsulotomy, A-scan biometry, IOL formulas, YAG laser capsulotomy, astigmatism control, and multifocal IOLs, Sir Ridley's dream has exceeded even his expectations. With all of these improvements in lens replacement surgery, we now have reliable phacorefractive approaches that rival, and even surpass, corneorefractive surgical procedures.

This text is intended to provide the latest information on refractive cataract surgery and to encourage the use of new technologies to improve patient satisfaction and to promote the advent of better methods to improve our effectiveness in this important new field.

FOREWORD

Vision is the most precious of the senses. Every human being desires high quality vision. But what is high quality vision? To me, it is the kind of vision I enjoyed for the first 40 years of my life; 20/15+ uncorrected in both eyes at distance and near, good color vision, a full field, and normal motility with stereopsis. I believe all our patients, whether young or old, desire this kind of vision. It is the dream of every cataract surgeon to provide this level of high quality vision to their surgical patients reproducibly and with a minimum morbidity.

Since 1949, when Harold Ridley, MD and José Barraquer, MD pioneered, respectively, the fields of intraocular lens implantation and corneal refractive surgery, a multitude of brilliant surgeons and scientists have collaborated to develop a body of knowledge, technology, and clinical skills which when combined bring the goal of high quality uncorrected vision closer to reality for the postoperative cataract patient. The marriage of two disciplines, cataract and lens implant surgery with refractive surgery, has in the past 20 years given birth to a new category of ophthalmic specialist: the refractive cataract surgeon. The refractive cataract surgeon and his/her scientific and industry collaborators are driven to provide their patients with the highest quality uncorrected distance and near vision possible.

In this book, editor R. Bruce Wallace III, MD has recruited an extraordinary group of authors to describe in detail the body of knowledge, technology, and surgical skills required to practice the art of refractive cataract surgery.

As to the future, why not better vision than I had at age 40 for me when I develop my cataract? I want the higher order aberrations in my optical system neutralized with a custom accommodating lens implant (or secondary laser enhancement) to give me 20/10+ at near and distance without correction after my cataract surgery. I believe if it can be dreamed it can be done!

Richard L. Lindstrom, MD

1

Evolution of Refractive Cataract Surgery

Robert H. Osher, MD

Refractive cataract surgery has become a well-defined and accepted philosophy by anterior segment surgeons. It simply means that there is a refractive goal or an intended target, necessitating careful presurgical planning and precise operative technique.

How this terminology evolved is less clear and probably reflects a number of major and minor advances in technology and technique. Clearly, the two men and their ideas that most significantly changed our specialty are Sir Harold Ridley and his introduction of the intraocular lens (IOL), and Dr. Charles Kelman's development of phacoemulsification. Without Sir Harold Ridley, cataract surgery would result in double-digit refractive errors with all of the drawbacks of aphakia. Dr. Kelman's absence would have sentenced us to never-ending incisions, innumerable sutures, and excessive amounts of astigmatism.

No doubt these were magnificent milestones along the path to emmetropia, which also included other breakthroughs such as the introduction of healon, which redefined the gentleness in which surgeons could operate inside the eye. Dr. Clifford Terry's surgical keratometer focused our attention on the astigmatic effect of the incision and the closure. The development of ultrasonography and the formulas devised for IOL calculation constituted a giant step forward, and we owe Drs. Cornelius Binkhorst, Kenneth Hoffer, Jack Holladay, Don Sanders, Jack Retzlaff, and Manus Kraff a debt of gratitude. We are also indebted to the industry for the evolution of phacoemulsification technology led by Alcon Surgical of Forth Worth, Texas. Dr. Thomas Mozzocco's concept of the foldable lens overcame the hurdle of wound size. The men who played an important role in the evolution of the incision include Dr. Richard Kratz's scleral tunnel, Dr. Jack Singer's frown, Dr. Michael McFarland's one-stitch closure, Dr. Paul Ernst's "no stitch" approach, and Dr. Howard Fine's venture into clear cornea.

My involvement, and perhaps the reason that I was invited to author this chapter, was with the introduction and teaching of several different refractive concepts aimed at the cataract surgeon.

Astigmatic Keratotomy Combined with Cataract Surgery

It may have seemed obvious that the refractive error following cataract surgery was the product of a sphere and an astigmatic component. Yet, when I completed my final year of Fellowship at the Bascom Palmer Eye Institute in Miami, the focus in cataract surgery was on induced rather than preexisting astigmatism. The world was obsessed with the Terry keratometer, the Kratz scleral tunnel, and suture types and closure techniques that attempted to minimize the amount of astigmatism created by routine cataract surgery.

All agreed that the newer ultrasound devices and the IOL formulas could provide the patient with wonderful vision following surgery. However, this approach was aimed at correcting the spherical component, rather than the astigmatic component, of the pseudophakic refractive error. The reduction of preexisting astigmatism at the time of cataract surgery was not considered in the 1970s and early 1980s, possibly because the standards by which we evaluated results were always measured several months after surgery and with spectacle correction. The time was never better for the birth of a new concept—the refractive cataract surgeon.

Between 1980 and 1982, I visited the operating rooms of surgeons who were investigating surgical techniques to correct naturally occurring astigmatism. Robert Martin, MD, George Tate, MD, Albert Neumann, MD, Robert Fenzl, MD, Spencer Thornton, MD, Lee Nordan, MD, and Clifford Terry, MD were all working in this area. I was so impressed and influenced by their innovative thinking that I began a study in 1983 addressing the correction of preexisting astigmatism by combining the use of transverse relaxing incisions with cataract surgery.[1] I realized that we could no longer accept the traditional standard of measuring success by the best spectacle-corrected vision several months following surgery. Instead, the definition had to center upon the uncorrected visual acuity.

My original technique consisted of placing a single, straight, corneal relaxing incision in the periphery, perpendicular to the steepest meridian at the conclusion of the operation, and then adding a second parallel incision around a conservative 7.0 to 10.5 mm diameter optical zone. My nomogram was quite simple (Table 1-1).[2]

Subsequently, William Maloney, MD introduced a more aggressive operation governed by intraoperative keratoscopy, in which he placed two pairs of transverse incisions prior to the phacoemulsification.[3] Other surgeons attempted to determine the effect of adding transverse corneal incisions to their cataract surgery by varying either the incision length (John Shepherd, MD),[4] number of incisions (Jim Davison, MD),[5] optical zone size (Gary Hall, MD),[6] or incision depth (James Gills, MD).[7] Dr. U. Merlin introduced arcuate incisions,[8] and Spencer Thornton, MD introduced a nomogram that emphasized principle variables (amount of astigmatism, age, intraocular pressure), and minor modifiers (corneal diameter and thickness).[9] Additional clinical and cadaver studies by Richard Lindstrom, MD confirmed the theory of coupling.[10]

While my patient selection criteria, operative technique, and clinical results have been presented at major meetings since 1984 and subsequently published, the key conclusions can be summarized as follows.[11-17]

1. Eighty-eight percent of eyes undergoing astigmatic keratotomy (AK) at the time of cataract surgery had a reduction of the preexisting astigmatism.
2. Optical zone size, consistent incision depth, and patient age were major factors influencing the outcome.

Table 1-1

Nomogram

Cylinder (Diopters)	Optical Zone (mm)
1.5	8.5
2.0	8.0
2.5	7.0 to 7.5
3.0	6.0 to 6.5
3.5	Two pairs: 6 and 8.5

3. The selection of the IOL power was not affected by the AK since the average pre-operative and postoperative Ks were equivalent.
4. Except for corneal abrasions, no complications were encountered.
5. All eyes in this study, except one with amblyopia, enjoyed a best-corrected visual acuity of 20/40 or better, comparable to our control population.
6. The uncorrected visual acuity was outstanding with 20/40 or better vision achieved in 76% without glasses. Only a fraction of these patients would have achieved this visual result had their cylinder not been reduced by AK.

Harsh criticism was not uncommon, and at the Cataract Congress in 1984 one of the leading surgeons in America equated the performance of this procedure with "playing God." Yet it has been satisfying to witness a slow but steady acceptance of the concept of combining cataract and astigmatic surgery, which has indeed stood the test of time.

EARLY UNCORRECTED VISION: A NEW STANDARD

In the late 1980s, I had the opportunity to present another controversial concept at major meetings in the United States and in Europe. The message was closely related to that of refractive cataract surgery; the presentation was entitled, "Early Uncorrected Vision: The New Gold Standard." The uncorrected portion of the title reflected the surgeon's accurate control of the spherical and astigmatic components of the pseudophakic refractive error. However, the early portion of the title challenged the accepted dogma that induced astigmatism had to decay. This observation was based upon the belief that "tight sutures" would create an initial cylinder incompatible with immediate clear vision. In fact, the surgeon was supposed to be concerned if the patient happened to see clearly when the patch was removed. I argued that it was not the sutures but rather the presence of corneal edema that mimicked the effect of tight sutures. My contention was simple: if we could modify the method of cataract surgery in order to avoid a swollen cornea, then the early visual outcome would be both clear and, of equal importance, stable.

In order to achieve this result, the industry was issued a technical challenge: get rid of the preset limited responses of the phaco machine and instead allow the surgeon to choose his own settings. The technique of slow motion phacoemulsification was developed for the exquisite control of the intraocular environment. By reducing the parameters of aspiration rate, vacuum, ultrasound power, and infusion, the flow turbulence inside the eye was greatly diminished and the corneas appeared sparkling clear.

In 1986, I reported our efforts to achieve early uncorrected vision of 20/40 or better that was attained in 75% of patients upon removing their patch on the first postoperative day.[18] Moreover, both the uncorrected vision and the refractive error remained stable, and the concept of refractive cataract surgery continued to evolve.

HYPEROPIC LENSECTOMY

In 1987, I presented the first cases of hyperopic lensectomy to the American Society of Cataract and Refractive Surgery (ASCRS) and subsequently published these controversial cases in the *Audiovisual Journal of Cataract and Implant Surgery* in 1989[19] and elsewhere. [20-23] Several years before, Dr. Franco Verzella, MD of Italy, provoked interest in the removal of the clear crystalline lens as a treatment for high myopia.[24] However, the significant risk of retinal detachment dampened the enthusiasm for this refractive procedure and provided the basis of criticism.[25-27]

I began a study consisting of a small group of patients with high hyperopia who were contact lens intolerant and experienced job-related problems with their glasses. My original thinking was that clear lensectomy in a high hyperope was analogous to implanting a secondary intraocular lens into an aphakic eye. If we could justify the risk of surgery to allow selected aphakes to become deliriously happy, why not apply the same rationale to the high hyperope with contact lens intolerance? After all, the incidence of serious complications, such as retinal detachment, associated with lens extraction in the high myope was not comparable and small incision surgery utilizing phacoemulsification had elevated the safety and success of lens extraction to unprecedented levels.

Armed with these convictions, I initially operated on four eyes with hyperopia ranging between 7.5 and 11 diopters. The axial length measured 20.0 mm or less. The strength of the intraocular lens selected was between 31 and 37 diopters. The patients were fully informed and their surgical procedures were uncomplicated. Each patient was highly satisfied with his surgical outcome, but I was not. The intended refractive error was missed by as much as 4 diopters of residual hyperopia. One patient developed a swollen optic disc unassociated with any reduction in acuity, afferent pupil, or visual field defect. Fortunately, the disc edema was resolved after 5 months. As the size of the study was expanded, I became more comfortable operating on the small eye with a shallow anterior chamber that often had a tendency toward positive pressure. I also became more aware of the importance of selecting the accurate IOL power when the axial length was 21 mm or less. In addition to consulting with some of the leading experts who have published their formulas for IOL selection in short eyes (Drs. Kenneth J. Hoffer[28] and Jack Holladay[29]), we developed a database correlating axial length and an additive "fudge factor" necessary to achieve emmetropia from which the IOL could be selected empirically.

Other ophthalmic surgeons also experienced favorable results following clear lens extraction in hyperopic eyes, including a series published by Lyle and Jin,[30] Koch,[31] Siganos,[32,33] and Isfahani.[34,35] Virtually all agreed that accurate IOL selection and the availability of high-powered IOLs were challenges. Piggybacking lenses for high hyperopia was introduced by Johnny Gayton, MD,[36] but the long-term safety has been questioned by later complications, such as the development of opacification between adherent lenses.[37] More recently, there is excitement about phakic implantation, but again, long-term safety is of the utmost importance. Yet, with respect to hyperopic lensectomy, the indications for surgical intervention were sound, each patient was happy, and the operation has earned the respect of cataract surgeons worldwide.

FINAL THOUGHTS

As we enter the new millennium, refractive cataract surgery has become an accepted concept around the planet. In retrospect, my small role was often to shoulder the criticism that inevitably accompanies any new philosophical direction. Admittedly, it is quite satisfying to recall two decades ago the words of the president of the American Academy of Ophthalmology (AAO) who admonished, "Bobby, you're going to throw your entire career away if you venture into these dark alleys afar from the mainstream of ophthalmology." But during a fellowship with Lawton J. Smith, MD, a renowned and revered neuro-ophthalmologist, I learned a valuable lesson which should be passed along to every young physician: "The truth is not defined by the majority opinion!" Refractive cataract surgery is here to stay, having earned its rightful place in ophthalmology.

REFERENCES

1. Osher RH. Annual Meeting of the American Intraocular Implant Society; 1984.

2. Osher RH. Transverse astigmatic keratotomy combined with cataract surgery. In: Thompson KP, Waring GO, eds. *Contemporary Refractive Surgery—Ophthalmology Clinics of North America*. Philadelphia, Pa: WB Saunders Co; 1992:717-725.

3. Maloney WF. Refractive cataract replacement: a comprehensive approach to maximize refractive benefits of cataract extraction. Paper presented at the annual meeting of the American Society of Cataract and Refractive Surgery. Los Angeles; 1986.

4. Shepherd JR. Induced astigmatism in small incision surgery. *J Cataract Refract Surg*. 1989; 15:85-88.

5. Davison JA. Transverse astigmatic keratotomy combined with phacoemulsification and intraocular lens implantation. *J Cataract Refract Surg*. 1989;15:38-44.

6. Hall GW, Campion M, Sorenson CM, et al. Reduction of corneal astigmatism at cataract surgery. *J Cataract Refract Surg*. 1991;17:407-414.

7. Gills JP. Relaxing incisions reduce postop astigmatism. *Ophthalmology Times*. 1991; Nov: 11.

8. Merlin U. Corneal keratotomy procedure for congenital astigmatism. *J Refract Surg*. 1987; 3:92-97.

9. Thornton SP. Theory behind corneal relaxing incisions/Thornton nomogram. In: Gills JP, Martin RG, Sanders DR, eds. *Sutureless Cataract Surgery*. Thorofare, NJ: SLACK Incorporated; 1992:123-144.

10. Lindstrom RL, Lindquist TD. Surgical correction of postoperative astigmatism. *Cornea*. 1988;7:138-148.

11. Osher RH. Presented at the annual meeting of the American Intraocular Implant Society; 1984.

12. Osher RH. Astigmatic keratotomy and cataract surgery. Presented at the annual meeting of the United Kingdom Intraocular Implant Society. Guernsey, England; 1985.

13. Osher RH. Combined cataract and astigmatism surgery. Presented at the Welsh Cataract Congress. Houston, Tex; 1986.

14. Osher RH. Combined cataract and astigmatism surgery: The use of relaxing keratotomy. Paper presented at the American International IOL Congress. Boston, Mass; 1985.

15. Osher RH. Paired transverse relaxing keratotomy: a combined technique for reducing astigmatism. *J Cataract Refract Surg*. 1989;15:30-37.

16. Osher RH. Relaxing keratotomy: an effective technique for reducing astigmatism at the time of cataract surgery. Presented at the annual meeting of the American Society of Cataract and Refractive Surgery. Los Angeles; 1986.

17. Osher RH. Transverse relaxing keratotomy: a combined procedure with cataract surgery for the reduction of astigmatism. Paper presented at the annual meeting of the American Academy of Ophthalmology. Atlanta; 1990.

18. Osher RH. Early uncorrected vision following cataract surgery: a new standard. Paper presented at the European Intraocular Implant lens Council. Zurich, Switzerland;1989.

19. Osher RH. Controversies in cataract surgery. *Audiovisual Journal of Cataract & Implant Surgery*. 1989;5(3).

20. Osher RH. Discussant. Management of patients with high ametropia who seek refractive surgical correction. *Eur J Implant Ref Surg*. 1994;6:298-299.

21. Osher RH. Clear lens extraction. Letter. *J Cataract Refract Surg*. 1994;20:674.

22. Osher RH. Hyperopic lensectomy: an update. Paper presented at the American Academy of Ophthalmology Annual Meeting. San Francisco; 1997.

23. Osher RH. Clear lensectomy. In: Fine IH, ed. *Clear Corneal Lens Surgery*. Thorofare, NJ; SLACK Incorporated; 1999:281-285.

24. Verzella F. Refractive surgery of the lens in high myopes. *Refract Corneal Surg*. 1990;6:273-275.

25. Lindstrom RL. Refractive surgery for the high myope: controversy and concern. Editorial. *J Refract Surg*. 1987;3:77-78.

26. Lindstrom RL. Ophthalmologic debate: is it reasonable to remove a healthy lens to improve vision? *JAMA*. 1987;257:2005.

27. Goldberg MF. Clear lens extraction for axial myopia: an appraisal. *Ophthalmology*. 1992;99 (suppl):108.

28. Hoffer KJ. The Hoffer Q formula: a comparison of theoretic and regression formulas. *J Cataract Refract Surg*. 1993;19:700-712.

29. Holladay JT, Gills JP, Leidlein J, Cherchio M. Achieving emmetropia in extremely short eyes with two piggyback posterior chamber intraocular lenses. *Ophthalmology*. 1996;103:1118-1123.

30. Lyle WA, Jin GJC. Clear lens extraction for the correction of high refractive error. *J Cataract Refract Surg*. 1994;20:273-276.

31. Koch P. Clear lensectomy for hyperopia. Paper presented at the American Society of Cataract and Refractive Surgery meeting. Seattle, Wash; 1993.

32. Siganos DS, Siganos CS, Pallikaris IG. Clear lens extraction and intraocular lens implantation in normally sighted hyperopia eyes. *J Refract Corneal Surg*. 1994;10:117-121.

33. Siganos DS, Pallikaris IG, Siganos CS. Clear lensectomy and intraocular lens implantation in normally sighted highly hyperopic eyes: 3-year follow-up. *Eur J Implant Ref Surg*. 1995;7:128-133.

34. Isfahani AHK, Salz JJ. Clear lens extraction with intraocular lens implantation for the correction of hyperopia. In: Sher N, ed. *Surgery for Hyperopia and Presbyopia*. Baltimore, Md: Williams & Wilkins; 1997.

35. Isfahani AM, Panglinan R, Shah S, et al. Surgical correction of hyperopia. In: Abbott R, Hwang D, eds. *Refractive Surgery—Ophthalmology Clinics of North America*. Philadelphia, Pa: WB Saunders Co; 1997.

36. Gayton JL, Sanders VN. Implanting two posterior chamber lenses in a case of microphthalmos. *J Cataract Refract Surg.* 1993;19:776-777.

37. Gayton JL, Bosc JM, Cohen JS, et al. Piggyback complications. *Video Journal of Cataract and Refractive Surgery*. 1999;15(2).

2 Ocular Biometry for IOL Calculations

Cynthia J. Kendall, BMET, RDMS, ROUB

INTRODUCTION

Twenty years ago I became involved in ultrasound for ophthalmology. At that time, not all surgeons performed preoperative biometry measurements prior to cataract removal and intraocular lens (IOL) implantation. Some used the clinical history method or looked up IOL powers on charts and tables using keratometry measurements and assumed pre-cataract refraction. The preoperative refraction (hopefully not including cataract induced changes) and the average keratometry reading were charted. Needless to say, accurate results were not obtained as often as desired. However, once a surgeon made the decision to begin measuring the axial length with ultrasound, surgery was often postponed until the instrument became available and the techniques of obtaining measurements could be learned. When interpretations of echo pattern subtleties and measurement caliper positions were understood, the quality of postoperative refractions improved.

IOL formulas have now moved into the fourth generation, incorporating both theoretical aspects and regression analysis. Surgical techniques are remarkably more advanced today, as are IOL manufacturing technologies. Along with these refinements come increased patient expectations and the need to perform preoperative measurements as accurately as possible. Over the years, everyone involved in producing a desirable postoperative refraction has made significant improvements.

A-scan Exam Techniques

The first method for performing axial length biometry was immersion, sometimes called the "water bath" technique. The primary advantage of this technique is its ability to obtain accurate data independent of the examiner. The goal of every diagnostician is to obtain accurate data from a patient without interfering with the data during the process. Since the immersion technique does not involve touching the cornea, the opportunity exists to observe and measure the truest possible axial length.

As the number of personnel performing scans increased, a somewhat simpler method became popular. This involved attaching the immersion shell directly to the A-scan probe and placing a tiny membrane over the end to contain the fluid. These were called water-filled probes and were used for many years. The primary disadvantage of this method was that the physicians and technicians had to make certain there were no air bubbles remaining in the probe after filling. A small 1 mm air bubble up against the probe tip membrane, and therefore in the pathway of the sound, could be responsible for a 3 diopter (D) postoperative refractive error.

In the mid 1980s, more technicians and residents were performing preoperative testing and the water-filled probe was thought to be too much trouble. The "solid" A-scan probe was then introduced. This probe eliminated the trouble of filling and avoiding air bubbles, but it increased the problem of corneal compression, also evident in the applanation technique of the water-filled probe.

Corneal Compression

Corneal compression[2] is the inadvertent shortening of axial length as a result of pressure from the A-scan probe in the contact technique. This is a result of touching the delicate cornea with a hard probe. Even with a gentle hand-held technique, or properly balanced tonometer or applanation device, compression may still occur.

It has been my observation that patients with steep corneas and/or low intraocular pressure (IOP) are more likely to demonstrate compressibility than do patients with normal corneal curvatures and IOP. Due to these and other unpredictable situations, performing contact A-scan biometry requires the examiner to extensively repeat measurements to assure that minimum pressure was applied to the eye. In instruments that produce a separate anterior chamber depth (ACD) measurement, observing changes in this value helps to monitor the amount of pressure. However, even with great attention and care, corneal compression may still occur. Compression of the cornea will produce a measurement shorter than it should be. This causes the IOL calculation formula to predict a stronger lens than is really needed, producing a degree of postoperative myopia.

For example, two contact measurements of an eye produced from valid echo patterns are 23.50 with ACD of 3.0 and 23.70 with ACD of 3.20. The thought should be that the first measurement of 23.50 includes some amount of compression. The rule in contact scans is to choose the longest reproducible axial length produced by a valid A-scan echo pattern having the deepest anterior chamber and the smoothest, tallest retinal echo edge. The scan must be repeated in order for the doctor to be confident that the measurement was obtained with the least corneal compression.

Compression was a factor even with water-filled probes, but it was lessened somewhat by the fact that the delicate latex membrane could conform to the cornea, making it a little easier to make gentle, complete contact. The solid probe, unfortunately, increases the likelihood of corneal compression, adding to this problem. People began to mount the A-scan probe in the tonometer portion of the slit lamp without completely understanding how to balance the delicate mechanism so as to minimize compression.

Coming Full Circle

Now, at the beginning of a new century, we have come full circle to the realization that the immersion method for performing scans produces the most reliable measurements with the least interference by the examiner. Therefore, it offers the benefit of consistently accurate results independent of the examiner. I am confident that after only a few patients you will see for yourself just how remarkable the immersion technique is. It is incredibly satisfying to observe the repetition of a measurement within a few hundredths of a millimeter. Once learned, results from the immersion technique are obtained more quickly than contact. The contact method requires the examiner to obtain many more measurements, looking for the best retinal echo, and to minimize corneal compression, the deepest ACD.

Patient Expectations

Patients today are more educated than ever before. They are doing their homework and speaking with others about what to expect from cataract surgery with IOL implantation. Monofocal technology has led researchers to meet the obvious need for the next step, multifocal IOL technology. With this refinement comes the need for refinement in every other possible area of influence. My motto has always been "everything can be improved." The desire to improve will always lead us to focus our thoughts on each and every step to see what can be done better. Our patients demand the best possible vision we can provide, and they deserve our full attention to detail.

A-Scan Basics

The "A" in A-scan stands for amplitude. A-scans are one-dimensional images in which echo strengths are displayed as vertical deflections, or "spikes" of varying heights, on a display screen. We interpret A-scan echoes in terms of their position and amplitude (height) on the display. There are several factors that control what makes an echo spike tall or short, good or bad.

Perpendicularity

The primary reason an echo is tall is because the sound beam is directed in a perpendicular fashion toward an interface between different ocular tissues. Just as a light beam reflects off a smooth surface, the sound beam is reflected as well. Imagine standing in front of a mirror and shining a flashlight beam straight ahead into the mirror. The reflected light would be so bright that you wouldn't be able to keep your eyes open. But, if the beam is tilted just a little, so that the angle is not exactly perpendicular to the mirror, the light will be reflected away from your eyes and into a different part of the room. The same idea holds true for sound beams. They are more difficult to understand because they are invisible, but if you try to imagine the sound beam as a light beam, it might help to anticipate its behavior. If a sound beam is not perpendicular to an ocular structure, an echo is produced but it will be reflected away from the probe. This results in a short or nonexistent echo on the screen. The tiny ophthalmic ultrasound probe is both the sender and receiver of sound. It must be very carefully positioned so that it may both "speak" and "hear" the echo when it returns.

Interfaces

An interface is the place where two different tissues meet. When the tissues are very different from each other, and the sound beam strikes the interface perpendicularly, a strong echo will be returned to the probe to be displayed on the screen as a tall spike.

Conversely, when two tissues at an interface are similar to each other, even if the sound beam is perpendicular, only a small echo will be returned to the probe and displayed on the screen as a small spike.

Surfaces

A third aspect to be considered regarding interfaces is their smoothness or roughness. Even when we know that a retinal echo should "always" be tall with a smooth leading edge, sometimes there is nothing we can do to produce the "correct" echo. This might be a case in which an underlying pathology is present. Macular diseases such as edema or age-related macular degeneration (ARMD), epiretinal membranes, and staphylomas where the macula might lie on a slope, are all situations in which the classic retinal echo may not be displayed.

As examiners, it is our job to do everything in our power to produce the correct echo pattern, and when we cannot do that we must properly document and report our findings to all who are involved in the treatment decisions for the patient.

Velocities and Measurements

An ultrasound beam travels through an eye, reflecting some of its energy each time an interface is encountered. The instrument measures the time required for a pulse of sound to travel to and from an interface, and divides the number in half, obtaining the one-way travel time. The assumed speed of sound for each ocular tissue type is applied and the distance in millimeters is then displayed on the screen for the examiner to see.

The speed of sound varies depending upon the tissue through which it travels. In aqueous and vitreous, for example, it is 1532 meters per second (m/s), while the speed of sound in the crystalline lens is 1641 m/s. This difference makes it important to know what kind of eye is to be measured—phakic, aphakic, or pseudophakic— so that the proper setting on the ultrasound instrument may be used. Knowing how an instrument arrives at a measurement will allow a manual correction to be made if the eye is inadvertently scanned in an incorrect mode. Ratios may be used to "undo" the measurement from the wrong velocity mode and convert it to a correct measurement without reexamining the patient. Understanding the concept of ultrasound velocities and how they affect the measurement opens the door to diagnosing difficult scan patterns.

Velocities of Sound in the Eye

- 1532 aqueous and vitreous
- 1641 crystalline lens
- 980 silicone oil

Electronic Calipers or Gates

Hand-in-hand with velocities is the discussion of electronic calipers, or gates as they are often called. For an instrument to measure accurately, it must detect which echo is to be measured. This is done with an electronic marker of some type—a line, dot, arrow, etc—displayed on the screen. Some calipers actually touch the echo being measured, while others are underneath or to the left of the echo. How they are displayed is not as important as understanding how they work. If the gates are positioned on an incorrect echo, an incorrect measurement will result. Interpretation of echo patterns, velocities, and caliper positions will guide the examiner to the correct answer.

SCAN COMPARISONS

A contact or immersion A-scan will produce the same essential echoes. The difference is that in the immersion technique, the probe tip echo is separated from the corneal echo. In the contact technique, where the probe makes contact with the cornea, these two echoes merge into one strong echo spike. In the immersion technique, where the probe is separated from and does not actually touch the cornea, the echo from the probe tip and the corneal echoes are clearly separated on the display.

Remember the three things that affect quality of any echo—perpendicularity, type of interface, and texture. No matter which exam technique is used or which eye type is being scanned, in order to obtain a tall echo in A-scan, the sound beam must be perpendicular to a smooth interface.

Each interface between dissimilar tissues will produce an echo. Think about where the sound beam needs to be directed in order to obtain a valid, accurate measurement. If unexpected echoes appear in the scan, discover what could have produced them. Does the patient have asteroid hyalosis or a posterior vitreous detachment (PVD)?

Normal

Measurements should be evaluated for how normal they are in general, their similarity to the fellow eye, and correlation with patient history. Over the years, thousands of scans have been evaluated to arrive at the same conclusion: the average axial eye length is approximately 23.50 mm.[3] Shorter eyes tend to be hyperopic and longer ones myopic. Between eyes, measurements should be within 0.3 mm unless clinical history explains the difference.[4]

If a patient with otherwise normal vision produces a measurement of 15 or 30 mm, there should be great suspicion. Somewhere, something is incorrect and evaluation of the echo patterns, measuring gates, and velocities should provide the answer. More information on troubleshooting appears later in this chapter.

Averaging

Once several scans have been obtained and stored, many people like to average them. It can be comforting to see a measurement that is the result of an average of many scans. However, caution must be observed here. If the averaging program in the A-scan instrument arbitrarily removes the longest and shortest measurement, thus averaging the remaining ones, it could very well be that the most correct value (the longest measurement) was discarded. The average of a series of numbers is only as accurate as the numbers used to create the average. Having a "low standard deviation" factor associated with an averaged number doesn't help either. This only means that the measurements used in the average were similar, not necessarily correct. Repeating a mistake is what we are trying to avoid; being accurate is what we are trying to achieve. My philosophy is that if the measurement is correct, one should be able to recreate both the scan and the measurement. When measurements are consistently within 0.05 mm to 0.10 mm, the need for averaging is eliminated.

Manual Mode

Most biometry instruments have a manual mode. The advantage of a manual mode is that the examiner may dynamically scan the eye, looking for the best echo pattern that the eye is capable of producing. Also, some instruments have a continuous display of axial length measurements for review during active scanning. This is the preferred method for most scans, contact or immersion, but especially required for immersion.

Automatic Mode

In the automatic mode, control of echo pattern interpretation is relinquished to the software algorithms inside the instrument. Sometimes they are quite good at selecting correct patterns, but other times they are not. An instrument does not make a better decision than a human about what constitutes a valid scan pattern. But, in situations with uncooperative patients, the automatic mode may be useful, as it will often acquire an image more quickly. An automatically frozen scan may be the best that can be achieved under special conditions.

No matter which mode is used, you must evaluate each and every frozen scan to see if you approve. If so, keep the scan. If not, delete it and keep trying. Remember, just because an instrument "beeps" that the scan is correct, never accept it until you have interpreted the pattern, calipers, and velocity setting.

Contact Technique

In the contact or applanation method, the first echo displayed on the screen is a combination of the probe tip and the corneal echoes. Since the probe tip is in contact with the cornea, echoes from the two cannot be separated. The first echo of a contact axial length A-scan is usually referred to as the cornea spike, although we now understand that it includes the probe tip echo as well. Diligent attention must always be applied to interpretation of echo patterns and corneal compression.

If the hand-held technique must be used for a special case, recline the patient so that the examiner has more hand and arm support. This may prove helpful for minimizing corneal compression and is more comfortable for both the patient and examiner.

In the slit lamp mounted applanation technique, balance the tonometer each time the probe is mounted. Before the patient exam, test the balance to verify that gentle yet sufficient pressure is maintained with corneal contact. Support the cable with a rubber band attached to the wire and to one of the oculars. This will help in two ways: (1) prevent damage to the wire and the tonometer mechanism from an inadvertent pull on the cable, and (2) reduce interference in balancing the tonometer by the weight of the A-scan probe cable.

Immersion Technique

In the immersion method, only fluid touches the cornea.[5] The probe tip is immersed into the mini water bath of liquid. The water bath is called a scleral shell, or immersion shell. It is placed on the anesthetized conjunctiva and filled with liquid. The kinder the fluid, the happier the patient. Thick methylcellulose, while it doesn't leak, can irritate many patients. Whenever possible, use a tear-like solution for greater patient comfort and cooperation. Explain to the patient that he/she will feel a cool liquid on his/her eye.

The probe tip echo maintains its stationary position on the left of the display screen. The anterior and posterior corneal surfaces will appear as a double-peaked echo to the right of the probe tip echo. The distance between them is determined by the amount of fluid in the shell and how deep the probe is suspended in the fluid. Two commonly used designs of scleral shells are Hansen and Prager.

Hansen shells are made by Hansen Ophthalmic Development Labs in Iowa City, Iowa. They make a set of shells in various diameters between 16 mm (for pediatric use) and 24 mm. The most popular sizes are 18 and 20 mm. The examiner holds the shell with one hand, while the probe is suspended in the fluid and directed toward the eye with the other hand. The advantages of the Hansen shell are its light weight, crystal clear plastic for ease of view, and choice of sizes. Disadvantages of the shell are that it requires a more steady hand, which can be challenging for beginners to master. It is often filled with methylcellulose to avoid leaks. However, methylcellulose is not only expensive, it is not always well tolerated by patients. It must be thoroughly rinsed from the eye to avoid blurring vision.

Thomas Prager, PhD approached the situation in a different way. Over the years, he has refined an idea to mount the A-scan probe into the shell so that they operate as a single unit. Once the shell/probe assembly is placed under the lids, saline is injected into the shell to fill the space between the cornea and the probe. The advantages of the Prager shell are that the corneal echoes appear in the same place on the screen all the time, it requires a less steady hand, can be performed using only one hand, and saline is more comfortable for the patient. Disadvantages include a little difficulty in visualizing the fluid level because the plastic is not completely clear, the slightly larger overall size, and its current availability in only one size.

ECHO INTERPRETATION

The keys to open the door of echo interpretation are found in understanding ultrasound principles and instrumentation. As long as you know the velocity at which measurements were made and can see the calipers or gates, you can make sense of the echo pattern and measurements. With these tools, any echo pattern from any instrument may be interpreted. An A-scan echo is evaluated in terms of its position within the echo pattern, height, smoothness of the leading edge, and sharpness of its intersection with the baseline.

If only one echo is obtained from the retina, with no other echoes after it, this indicates that the sound beam was directed toward the optic disc, not the macula.[6] If you think about what the sound beam is doing when it is directed toward the disc, you can see that there are no posterior structures to which the beam can be perpendicular. The sound beam is parallel to the optic nerve tissue; therefore, no echo is displayed.

However, when directed toward the macula, the beam will be perpendicular to the underlying structures of sclera and orbital fat, producing a characteristic echo complex.

What to Look For in a Phakic Scan

In an eye with a crystalline lens, whether cataractous or not, look for these echoes:
1. Tall echo from the cornea (one echo in contact technique and a double-peaked echo in immersion)
2. Tall echo from anterior lens capsule
3. Medium to tall echo from posterior lens capsule
4. Tall, sharply rising retinal echo with a perfect 90-degree angle between the bottom of the echo and where it connects with the baseline
5. Medium to tall echo from the sclera
6. Medium to low echoes from the orbital fat[7]

Since a cataractous lens is not a completely uniform tissue, small and sometimes even large interfaces may be present. These interfaces may be displayed as extra echoes between the anterior and posterior lens surfaces. The echoes may be disregarded unless the measuring gates are attached to them, producing an incorrectly small lens thickness measurement. In the case of an instrument that uses independent velocities instead of an average velocity, gates triggering on cataractous echoes could also impact the accuracy of the total length due to the velocity difference within the lens material.

What to Look For in an Aphakic Scan

Sometimes an echo is produced from the intact posterior capsule, other times not, so don't be alarmed by the presence of an echo where the lens used to be. Pay extra attention to the retina/sclera/orbit complex of echoes, as there are no lens echoes to additionally guide your evaluation of the scan pattern.

Look for these echoes in an aphakic scan:
1. Tall echo from the cornea (one echo in contact technique and a double-peaked echo in immersion)
2. Occasional echo from lens capsule
3. Tall, sharply rising echo from the retina with a perfect 90-degree angle at the bottom of the echo where it connects with the baseline
4. Medium to tall echo from the sclera
5. Medium to low echoes from the orbital fat

What to Look For in a Pseudophakic Scan

Pseudophakic A-scans are always a challenge. Often the reverberation echoes in polymethylmethacrylate (PMMA) lenses startle us, or we have no idea what IOL material is inside the patient's eye and so do not know what pseudophakic setting to use. PMMA acrylic and silicone IOLs vary in their ultrasound velocities and in the thickness of each implant. The thickness of the IOL will affect the measurement. Values used to compensate for the velocity within an IOL are based upon an average power and thickness. Some newer IOL designs have less variance of lens thickness depending upon the power.

One of the simplest methods to measure an eye with an unknown IOL was described by Jack T. Holladay, MD.[8] Since a pseudophakic eye is about 98% aqueous and vitreous, first measure it in the aphakic mode with the velocity of 1532 m/s. The measured length is then modified depending upon the IOL material. Recently, it has been noted that some silicone IOLs do not need as much correction as was originally proposed. For PMMA lenses, the aphakic measurement is increased by 0.44 mm. For acrylic lenses, the apha-kic measurement is increased by 0.24 mm. In eyes with silicone IOLs the aphakic meas-urement must be decreased by 0.44 to 0.84 mm depending upon the material and design. When the IOL material is not known, measure as aphakic, add or subtract all the values, and compare with the fellow eye whenever possible.

Look for these echoes in a pseudophakic scan:

1. Tall echo from the cornea (one echo in the contact technique and a double-peaked echo in immersion)
2. Tall echoes from the anterior IOL surface with varying amount of "reverberation" echoes that are characteristic of PMMA and are much fewer with other IOL mate-rials
3. Tall, sharply rising echo from the retina with a perfect 90-degree angle at the bot-tom of the echo where it connects with the baseline
4. Medium to tall echo from the sclera
5. Medium to low echoes from the orbital fat

Silicone Oil in the Vitreous

Although a patient with silicone oil in the vitreous is most likely not a good candidate for a multifocal IOL, special attention is required in order to produce a valid measure-ment.

Look for these echoes in an eye filled with silicone oil:

1. Tall echo from the cornea (one echo in the contact technique and a double-peaked echo in the immersion method)
2. Tall echoes from both the anterior and posterior lens capsules
3. Multiple reverberation echoes following the posterior lens
4. Difficult to get tall, sharply rising echo from the retina with a perfect 90-degree angle at the bottom of the echo at the point where it connects with the baseline
5. Short or nonexistent echo from the sclera

The biometer's retina gate may have to be moved to the right in order to accommo-date the false long measurement produced by eyes with silicone oil. Since the velocity in silicone oil is so slow, 980 m/s, the sound beam takes longer to reach the retina and return. The measurement produced by a standard biometer may be used to recalculate the axial length in these patients. Subtract the ACD and lens thickness from the total length, leaving the vitreous/oil measurement. Recalculate this "vitreous" length by multi-plying it by the correct silicone oil velocity of 980 m/s.

TROUBLESHOOTING

When troubleshooting pre- or postoperatively, look for the simple things about the A-scan first.

- Is the echo pattern correct?
- Is the mode/velocity selection on the biometer correct?
- Are the measuring calipers in their correct positions?
- How does the measurement compare with the fellow eye?
- How does the measurement correlate with the patient's history?

In the case of a preoperative uncertainty, try to postpone surgery until answers can be found. Ask for assistance. There are many colleagues throughout the world who would gladly help to evaluate scan patterns. Try faxing or e-mailing images for another opinion. In the long run, knowledge will be gained and the patient, as well as future patients, will experience an optimal result.

Also important in the case of an undesirable postoperative result is to check all other input data of the IOL formula for accuracy. Specifically, monitor the postoperative IOL position. An IOL that ends up more anteriorly than predicted will produce myopia. Conversely, an IOL that has a postoperative position more posteriorly than anticipated will produce hyperopia.

Look for evidence of tolerance stacking. This occurs when small tolerances inherent in each piece of data stack up in one direction. This means that a +0.25 diopter (D) error in the keratometer (K) readings, a +0.25D tolerance on the IOL power, a +0.25D error from a slightly too long axial length, and a +0.25D effect from the IOL position being deeper than anticipated, together equal a 1D cumulative error. Careful evaluation of all the factors involved usually results in resolving the question.

The best method to ensure success is for you and your staff to develop your own protocol to verify that input data are accurate. Take a step back, look at the whole picture, and ask yourself, "Does this make sense?" Have patience with your patients.

REFERENCES

1.   Binkhorst RD. The accuracy of ultrasonic measurement of the axial length of the eye. *Ophthalmic Surgery*. 1981;12:363-365.

2.   Shammas HJ. A comparison of immersion and contact techniques for axial length measurements. *American Intraocular Implant Society Journal*. 1984;10:444-447.

3.   Holladay JT, Prager TC, Chandler TY, Musgrove KH. A three-part system for refining intraocular lens power calculations. *J Cataract Refractive Surgery*. 1988;14:17-24.

4.   Byrne SF. *A-Scan Axial Eye Length Measurements*. Mars Hill, NC: Grove Park Publishers; 1995;3:41-46.

5.   Byrne SF. *A-scan Axial Eye Length Measurements*. Mars Hill, NC: Grove Park Publishers; 1994;4:61-63.

6.   Kendall C. *Ophthalmic Echography*. Thorofare, NJ: SLACK Incorporated; 1990;4:67-70.

7.   Holladay JT, Prager TC. Accurate ultrasonic biometry in pseudophakia (letter). *American Journal of Ophthalmology*. 1993;115:536-537.

3 Optical Coherence Biometry

William P. Burnham, OD

THE CLINICAL PROBLEM

Precise measurement of eye parameters is critical in modern ophthalmology. In cataract surgery and refractive lensectomy, the measured axial length is the most significant component of the intraocular lens (IOL) power calculation, with a measurement error in axial length by acoustical A-scan ultrasound biometry being the leading cause of unplanned postoperative refractive error.[1] Inaccurate axial length measurements account for 54% of the errors in predicted refraction after IOL implantation.[1] This unplanned postoperative refractive error results from numerous sources of error in the ultrasound technique, which limit its best clinical accuracy to a range of approximately 0.10 to 0.12 mm.[2] These sources of error are technician dependent, originating primarily from improper examination techniques or incorrect instrument settings (Table 3-1). The end result of an axial length measurement error of 0.10 mm is a corresponding postoperative refractive error of 0.28 D.[1] Therefore, a skilled and knowledgeable biometrist is a prerequisite to obtain consistent and accurate measurements with the ultrasound technique. In addition to inaccuracy, there are other disadvantages in acoustical biometry. The procedure is an inconvenient and uncomfortable one for the patient, requiring a topical anesthetic. Corneal abrasion and transmission of infectious agents are significant complications of corneal contact in the ultrasound technique. Acoustical A-scan ultrasound biometry has proven to be an inaccurate axial length measurement technique for IOL power determination.

AN EMERGING SOLUTION

A solution to the limitations of acoustical A-scan ultrasound biometry is a new instrument called the Zeiss IOLMaster (Zeiss, Jena, Germany) (Figure 3-1). This optical coherence biometry device is a phenomenal breakthrough in both measurement technology

Table 3-1

Sources of Error in Acoustical Biometry

- Misalignment of the sound beam
- Inaccurate lens thickness measurement
- Improper gain setting
- Corneal compression (contact)
- Fluid bridge (contact)
- Inaccurate sound velocity
- Air bubble adherent to transducer (contact)
- Air bubble in fluid bath (immersion)

Figure 3-1. The Zeiss IOL-Master.

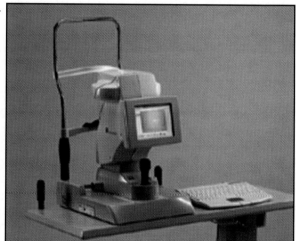

and patient care in the field of cataract surgery and refractive lensectomy. The IOLMaster by Carl Zeiss is the first noncontact, single-instrument system providing cataract and refractive surgeons with swift and accurate measurements of axial length, corneal curvature, and anterior chamber depth (ACD). The noncontact measurements of these parameters integrated into one device provides for a high level of patient comfort while increasing the efficiency of proper lens determination. Combining the measured values with the surgeon's personalized lens database, the IOLMaster calculates multiple IOL power implant options using known empirical or theoretical intraocular lens power formulas.

Patient expectation for functional uncorrected visual acuity and spectacle freedom after cataract or refractive surgery has increased. The IOLMaster offers the surgeon both the accuracy to reach postoperative refractive goals and the ability to increase practice efficiency.

IOLMaster Description

The IOLMaster consists of an integrated optical or measuring head, a power supply, an LCD screen, and a central processing unit (CPU). Within the optical head are the measurement components for determination of axial length, corneal curvature, and

ACD. The instrument base contains the power supply and CPU with interfaces. The LCD screen is used for observation and alignment of the patient's eye during measurement, as well as to display the measurement results. The IOLMaster is operated by using the keyboard with integrated mouse pad and the joystick of the instrument base. The software runs on Windows 95 and offers an intuitive graphic user interface.

IOLMaster Modes

The IOLMaster features three functional measurement modes and one IOL calculation mode. LCD screen buttons allow for easy transition between modes:
- Axial length
- Corneal curvature
- Anterior chamber depth
- IOL calculation

Advantages of the IOLMaster

Accuracy

- Precise axial length values are obtained along the visual axis on a range of eyes including high myopes, aphakes, pseudophakes, and silicone filled eyes
- Reliable and repeatable readings independent of technician technique

Practice Efficiency and Patient Flow

- Three measurements using one instrument reduces preparation and exam time
- Measure axial length, corneal curvature, and ACD on one eye in about a minute

Ease of Use

- No corneal applanation or pupil dilation
- Operational under all lighting conditions
- Detects right/left eye automatically
- Intuitive and familiar Windows interface
- Option of data transfer or printout

Patient Safety and Compliance

- No anesthetic required
- Quick and easy procedure
- Noncontact technique precludes corneal lesions and transmission of infectious agents

PARTIAL COHERENCE INTERFEROMETRY

The IOLMaster uses optical coherence biometry to measure the axial length of the human eye. Optical coherence biometry is noncontact in nature and is based on the principles of laser interferometry with partially coherent light, often termed partial coherence interferometry (PCI) (Figure 3-2). A laser diode emits light ($\lambda = 780$ nm) of short

Figure 3-2. Schematic of optical coherence biometry by Haigis and Fercher.

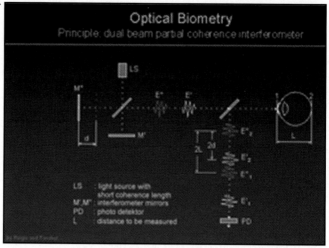

coherence length that is split up into two beams by a Michelson interferometer. Both beams illuminate the eye through a beam-splitting prism and reflect at both the cornea and retina. The light reflected by the cornea interferes with that reflected by the retina if the optical paths of both beams are equal. The interference is detected by a photodetector and the signals are amplified, filtered, and recorded as a function of the position of the interferometer mirror. Precise measurement of the interferometer mirror position enables the system to accurately determine the axial length as the path difference between the cornea and the retina. Axial length measurement with PCI has a precision more than 10 times better than that of ultrasound.[3] Comparing PCI to contact A-scan ultrasound, Drexler et al found PCI to result in a 27% improvement in the possible mean absolute error for postoperative refraction.[3]

OPTICAL COHERENCE BIOMETRY

The axial length measurement with the IOLMaster is accurate and reproducible. Optical coherence biometry with the IOLMaster is an automated, objective measurement of the axial length affected by none of the subjective error sources of acoustical A-scan ultrasound biometry. Measurement along the visual axis is ensured as the patient fixates on the light source, precluding a misalignment error produced by an off-axis posterior staphyloma. Furthermore, reliable and repeatable readings are obtained independent of operator technique. The preliminary finding of the accuracy achieved with the IOLMaster for axial length measurements in vivo is less than 0.05 mm. The actual accuracy may be better and further studies are being undertaken to quantify the exact accuracy of the IOLMaster. Haigis and Lege in Wuerzburg, Germany, found on 155 eyes an average standard deviation for five consecutive axial length measurements with the IOLMaster to be 0.023 mm ± 0.015 mm.[4]

Optical coherence biometry is a comfortable and safe procedure for patients. It is quickly and easily performed with the patient sitting upright in a manner similar to evaluation with the slit lamp (Figure 3-3). No anesthetic or dilation drops are required, and the technique precludes both corneal lesions and transmission of infectious agents. The total examination time required for five axial length measurements, corneal curvature readings, and anterior chamber depth readings is about 1 minute per eye.

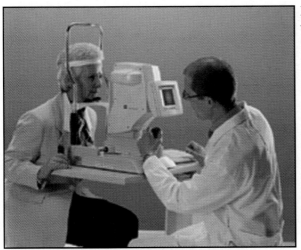

Figure 3-3. Examination setup with the IOLMaster.

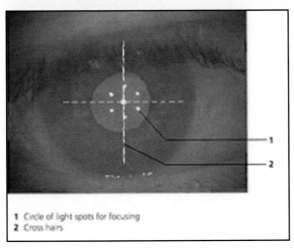

1 Circle of light spots for focusing
2 Cross hairs

Figure 3-4. Display image of the eye with correctly aligned instrument in overview mode.

IOLMASTER PRINCIPLES OF OPERATION

Axial Length Mode

Axial length alignment and measurement with the IOLMaster is simple. Starting with the low magnification of the overview mode, the operator focuses and superimposes the circle of lights over the display cross hair while the patient fixates on the yellow light source (Figure 3-4). The overview mode is for coarse alignment of the eye. The operator then presses the joystick button and the instrument switches to the axial length measurement mode. On activation of the axial length mode, the instrument automatically changes the magnification so that a smaller section of the eye becomes visible as well as a reflection of the alignment light and a vertical line. The patient is then asked to fixate on the red light source. On the display, a cross hair with a ring in the middle appears. The operator then aligns the instrument so that the vertical line is optimally focused, and the reflection of the alignment light at the same time appears focused within the ring of

Figure 3-5. Axial length alignment: 1. vertical line, 2. alignment light, 3. cross hair on display.

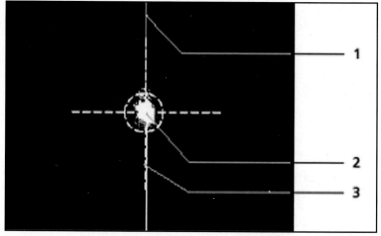

the cross hair (Figure 3-5). A push of the joystick button releases the measurement, which has an impulse duration of 0.5 seconds. It is recommended to take five measurements per eye. In order to protect the patient from excessive laser light, a maximum of 20 measurements per eye per day is permitted with the IOLMaster. For axial length technical data see Table 3-2.

Evaluation of Axial Length Measurements

The results of axial length measurements with the IOLMaster must be evaluated on the basis of the signal-to-noise ratio (SNR) and interpretation of the axial length graphs.

The instrument will automatically calculate the average of the axial length measurements provided that variation between the measurements and the mean of these measurements does not exceed $\pm$ 0.1 mm.

Signal-to-Noise Ratio (SNR)

The SNR is an indicator of the quality of the axial length measurement. The SNR is automatically assessed during the internal calculation of the axial length from the interference signal.

SNR Categories

- SNR > 2.0 = the measurement is valid
- SNR in the range of 1.6 to 2.0 = the measurement is borderline. These values are listed with an exclamation point after them to inform the operator that they are borderline (Figure 3-6). Accurate measurements can be determined by comparison with other values of the measurement series. It may occur that many or all measurements of a particular eye are borderline but still useful since they are in agreement with one another upon verification.
- SNR < 1.6 = the measurement is not usable (error). These measurements are listed as "Error" in the results column (Figure 3-7). This implies that the true measuring signal does not stand out from the noise.
- The SNR may be low for the following reasons:
  1. Dense medial opacity along the visual axis

Table 3-2

Technical Data of Axial Length Mode

Measuring range	14 to 39 mm
Accuracy on test eye	± 0.01 mm
Display resolution	0.01 mm
Reproducibility on eye	< ± 0.03mm
Wavelength	780 nm
Impulse duration	0.5 sec

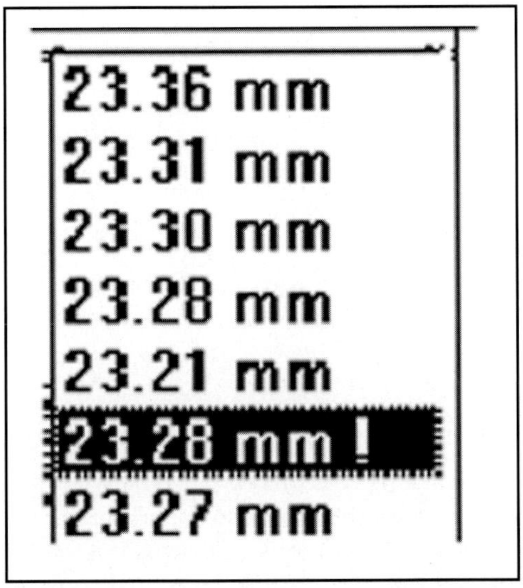

Figure 3-6. Borderline reading (SNR is between 1.6 and 2.0).

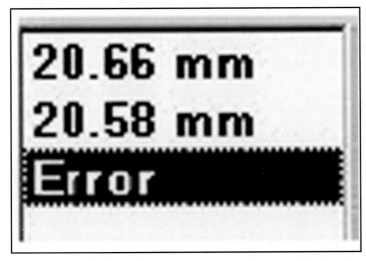

23.36 mm
23.31 mm
23.30 mm
23.28 mm
23.21 mm
23.28 mm !
23.27 mm

20.66 mm
20.58 mm
Error

Figure 3-7. Erroneous result (SNR < 1.6).

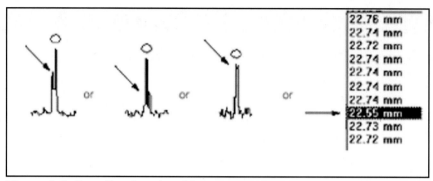

Figure 3-8. Broadband peaks with corresponding measurement variation.

2. Restless or poorly fixating patients
3. Patient blinks during measurement
4. Alignment error
5. Very high uncorrected myopia (> 6 D). (Note: try measuring through spectacles!)
6. Corneal scars
7. Retinal pathology

With these limitations, measurement may not be possible with the IOLMaster. Early analysis has found that these limitations can prevent an IOLMaster measurement in approximately 5% to 10% of patients.

Interpretation of the Axial Length Graph

Acoustical ultrasound biometry measures the axial length as that distance between the cornea and the inner limiting membrane (ILM) of the retina because sound waves are reflected at this retinal membrane. Optical coherence biometry with the IOLMaster measures the axial length as that distance between the cornea and the retinal pigment epithelium (RPE). To ensure that the measured axial length values obtained with the IOLMaster are compatible with those obtained acoustically, the IOLMaster system uses normative data to automatically adjust for the difference in distance between the ILM and the RPE. The displayed axial length values of the IOLMaster are thus directly comparable to those measured acoustically using the immersion technique.

It is very important to know that the correct axial length measurement with the IOLMaster must be such that the measuring cursor is placed at the RPE. Since the instrument places the cursor (and hence calculates the axial length) at the highest signal peak coming from the retina using automatic peak detection, it is important to verify that this is the RPE. Depending on the anatomical conditions of the measured eye, it may also happen that the measuring beam produces interference when being reflected at the ILM and/or the choroid. This would be indicated by broader peaks of the measuring curve with possible resultant variations of axial length data by approximately 0.15 to 0.35 mm in one measurement series (Figure 3-8). Only if the signal peak of these other structures is greater than that of the RPE will the measuring cursor be placed at them, and the axial length be computed incorrectly. These graphs may be evaluated between individual measurements in axial length mode or in post-measurement editing. Graph evaluation can be done with the help of the zoom function.

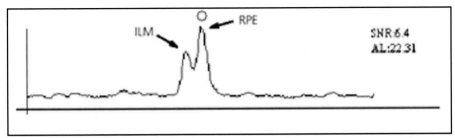

Figure 3-9. Double peak produced at the ILM (left) and RPE (right) (triple zoom).

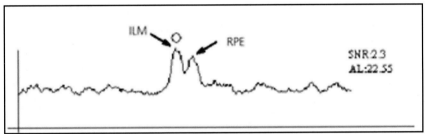

Figure 3-10. Signal curve with higher signal from ILM (left peak) (double zoom).

Signal Peak From the Inner Limiting Membrane (ILM)

Measuring light is often reflected at the ILM so that a double peak graph results. The corresponding ILM signal peak appears to the left of the signal peak for the RPE by a distance of about 0.15 to 0.35 mm (Figure 3-9). Usually, the signal peak produced by the ILM is smaller than that reflected by the RPE. In this case, the measuring cursor is placed at the signal peak of the RPE and the automatic algorithm finds the correct axial length. If the measuring cursor is placed at the ILM because its peak is higher than that of the RPE, it will produce an inaccurate axial length that is shorter by a value of 0.15 to 0.35 mm (Figure 3-10). Such individual measurements stand out by deviations in the range of 0.15 to 0.35 mm toward shorter axial lengths. Furthermore, this is the most likely reason that no average axial length value is generated for a measurement series. You may correct the measured value by manually moving the measuring cursor to the right to the smaller peak produced by the RPE or delete the reading. If you decide to manually move the measuring cursor, the measurement value will be permanently denoted by an asterisk indicating manipulation (Figure 3-11).

Signal Peak From the Choroid

In rare cases, it may happen that the measuring light is also reflected from the vessels of the choroid. The measuring peak produced by the choroid appears shifted toward longer axial lengths by approximately 0.15 to 0.25 mm from the peak of the RPE. When three signal peaks are present, it is important to know the corresponding structures and distances (Figure 3-12). It may occur in a triple peak presentation that the measuring cursor has been incorrectly placed at the ILM (Figure 3-13). After comparing all values for this eye, the measuring cursor must be moved manually to the middle and smaller peak

Figure 3-11. Manipulated measurement value.

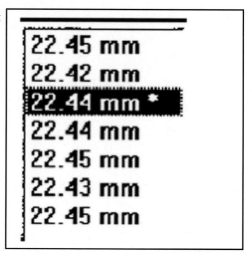

Figure 3-12. Triple peak with corresponding structures and distances.

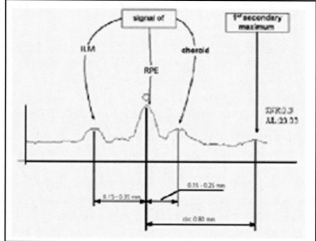

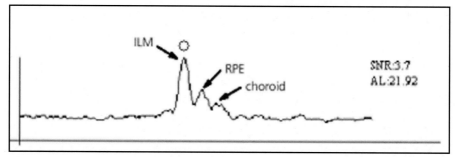

Figure 3-13. Triple peak with measuring cursor placed erroneously at ILM (double zoom).

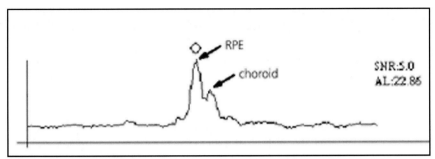

Figure 3-14. Double peak with RPE and choroidal spikes (double zoom).

produced by the RPE. A double peak graph produced by the RPE and choroid is also possible (Figure 3-14). This curve may only be evaluated correctly by viewing all measuring curves of this eye. Furthermore, this curve must be distinguished from double peaks produced by the ILM and RPE. It may be necessary to delete suspicious curves and take additional measurements (20 measurements are allowed per eye per day).

Personalization of Lens Constants

It is absolutely necessary to repersonalize the "lens constants" for use with the IOLMaster prior to applying its calculation values to determine an accurate IOL power. Refer to the literature and the publication of the authors of the IOL formulas regarding the personalization of constants. A side-by-side comparison of measurements with the IOLMaster against a surgeon's standard keratometric and ultrasonic axial length measurement techniques should be performed on approximately 50 eyes by each surgeon. It is important that traditional biometry methods be used to calculate all IOL powers until this personalizing of lens constants for the IOLMaster is satisfactorily completed. If proper lens constant personalization specific for this instrument is not performed, unwanted postoperative refractive errors are likely.

Corneal Curvature Mode

Central corneal curvature in diopters K, or radius of curvature in millimeters, is easily obtained with the integrated autokeratometer of the IOLMaster. The corneal curvature is determined by measuring the distance between six reflected infrared light images that are captured by a charge-coupled device (CCD) camera. After superimposing the six peripheral light sources with the green circular cross hair on the display, the measurement is released by pressing the joystick button (Figure 3-15). The measurement results are distance independent in a range of ± 2 mm. The displayed results are the average of five individual measurements taken within 0.5 seconds and include corneal curvature of the principal meridians with corresponding axes displayed in diopters K and millimeters, the dioptric difference between the principal meridians, and the refractive index (n) used to convert corneal radii into corneal refractive power in diopters. For autokeratometer technical data, see Table 3-3.

Table 3-3

Technical Data of the Autokeratometer

Measuring range diopters	33 to 67 D
Measuring range radii	5 to 10 mm
Astigmatism	≤ 10 D
Accuracy	± 0.05 mm
Display resolution	0.01 mm
Diameter of measuring area	< 3.0 mm

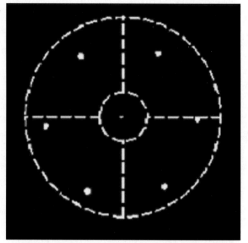

Figure 3-15. Alignment for corneal curvature measurement.

Anterior Chamber Depth Mode

The anterior chamber depth of the eye may be measured with the IOLMaster if desired. The ACD is measured as the distance between the optical sections of the cornea and the crystalline lens produced by lateral slit illumination of approximately 30 degrees to the optical axis. A CCD camera captures the image for processing. The lateral slit illumination flickers during measurement and always originates from the temporal field of the eye being measured. After alignment, the measurement is released by pushing the button on the joystick (Figure 3-16). The ACD measurement with the IOLMaster must be preceded by the keratometry measurement to obtain a reading. If K readings were not possible with the IOLMaster, they must be entered manually prior to the ACD measurement. For ACD measurement technical data, see Table 3-4.

IOL Calculation Mode

Prior to IOL calculation, you must first establish the surgeon-specific database by entering desired lens types and constants for each surgeon. The IOLMaster database can accommodate up to 20 surgeons, each having up to 20 desired IOLs with corresponding

Table 3-4

Technical Data of ACD Measurement

Measuring range	1.5 to 6.5 mm
Display resolution	0.01 mm

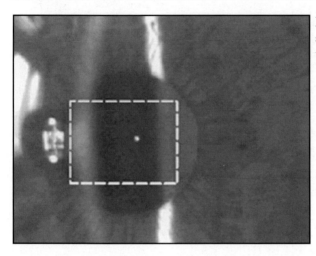

Figure 3-16. Alignment for anterior chamber depth measurement.

constants. After completion of the eye measurements, the results are automatically transferred to the IOL calculation page so that the surgeon can begin to calculate IOL powers to match his or her postoperative refractive requirements. The surgeon first selects the tab corresponding to the desired IOL calculation formula (Figure 3-17). The IOLMaster includes the following five integrated IOL calculation formulas: Haigis, Hoffer Q, Holladay, SRK II, and SRK/T. After choosing his or her name from the surgeon list box, the surgeon is able to access and select from his or her database up to four different IOLs for calculation. Recommended IOL powers are quickly generated after input of target refraction and a click on the "calculate IOL" button. The IOL power closest to the target refraction is located centrally in each column of selected lens types. This IOL power is highlighted on the printout of the IOL calculation page (Figure 3-18).

SUMMARY

Preoperative measurements with the Zeiss IOLMaster have many advantages compared to the conventional techniques of A-scan ultrasound biometry and keratometry. Improvements in accuracy, ease of use, and patient safety and compliance will have a very positive impact on the ophthalmological practice. Furthermore, enhanced practice efficiency and patient flow will be achieved through the use of the IOLMaster. Optical coherence biometry and the IOLMaster represent a technological advancement that enables surgeons to refine their postoperative refractive results to improve the quality of life of their patients.

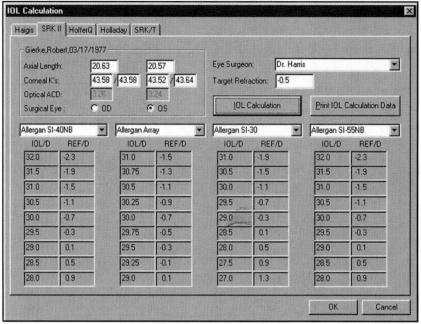

Figure 3-17. IOL Calculation mode.

REFERENCES

1. Olsen T. Sources of error in IOL power calculations. *J Cataract Refract Surg.* 1992;18(3):125-129.

2. Binkhorst RD. The accuracy of ultrasonic measurements of the axial eye length. *Ophthalmic Surg.* 1981;12:363-365.

3. Drexler W, Findl O, Menapace R. Partial coherence interferometry: a novel approach to biometry in cataract surgery. *Am J Ophthalmol.* 1998;126(4):524-534.

4. Haigis W, Lege BM. First experiences with a new optical biometry device. ESCRS Presentation. 1999; Vienna, Austria.

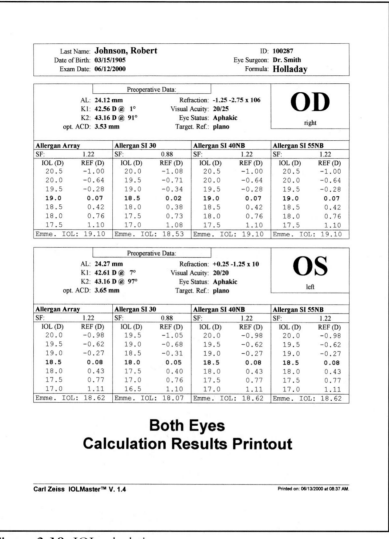

Last Name: **Johnson, Robert**	ID: **100287**
Date of Birth: **03/15/1905**	Eye Surgeon: **Dr. Smith**
Exam Date: **06/12/2000**	Formula: **Holladay**

Preoperative Data:

AL: **24.12 mm** Refraction: **-1.25 -2.75 x 106**
K1: **42.56 D @ 1°** Visual Acuity: **20/25**
K2: **43.16 D @ 91°** Eye Status: **Aphakic**
opt. ACD: **3.53 mm** Target. Ref.: **plano**

OD
right

Allergan Array		Allergan SI 30		Allergan SI 40NB		Allergan SI 55NB	
SF:	1.22	SF:	0.88	SF:	1.22	SF:	1.22
IOL (D)	REF (D)	IOL (D)	REF (D)	IOL (D)	REF (D)	IOL (D)	REF (D)
20.5	-1.00	20.0	-1.08	20.5	-1.00	20.5	-1.00
20.0	-0.64	19.5	-0.71	20.0	-0.64	20.0	-0.64
19.5	-0.28	19.0	-0.34	19.5	-0.28	19.5	-0.28
19.0	**0.07**	**18.5**	**0.02**	**19.0**	**0.07**	**19.0**	**0.07**
18.5	0.42	18.0	0.38	18.5	0.42	18.5	0.42
18.0	0.76	17.5	0.73	18.0	0.76	18.0	0.76
17.5	1.10	17.0	1.08	17.5	1.10	17.5	1.10
Emme. IOL: 19.10		Emme. IOL: 18.53		Emme. IOL: 19.10		Emme. IOL: 19.10	

Preoperative Data:

AL: **24.27 mm** Refraction: **+0.25 -1.25 x 10**
K1: **42.61 D @ 7°** Visual Acuity: **20/20**
K2: **43.16 D @ 97°** Eye Status: **Aphakic**
opt. ACD: **3.65 mm** Target. Ref.: **plano**

OS
left

Allergan Array		Allergan SI 30		Allergan SI 40NB		Allergan SI 55NB	
SF:	1.22	SF:	0.88	SF:	1.22	SF:	1.22
IOL (D)	REF (D)	IOL (D)	REF (D)	IOL (D)	REF (D)	IOL (D)	REF (D)
20.0	-0.98	19.5	-1.05	20.0	-0.98	20.0	-0.98
19.5	-0.62	19.0	-0.68	19.5	-0.62	19.5	-0.62
19.0	-0.27	18.5	-0.31	19.0	-0.27	19.0	-0.27
18.5	**0.08**	**18.0**	**0.05**	**18.5**	**0.08**	**18.5**	**0.08**
18.0	0.43	17.5	0.40	18.0	0.43	18.0	0.43
17.5	0.77	17.0	0.76	17.5	0.77	17.5	0.77
17.0	1.11	16.5	1.10	17.0	1.11	17.0	1.11
Emme. IOL: 18.62		Emme. IOL: 18.07		Emme. IOL: 18.62		Emme. IOL: 18.62	

Both Eyes
Calculation Results Printout

Carl Zeiss IOLMaster™ V. 1.4   Printed on: 06/13/2000 at 08:37 AM.

Figure 3-18. IOL calculation page.

4 Important Considerations for IOL Calculations

Kenneth J. Hoffer, MD

INTRODUCTION

The calculation of intraocular lens (IOL) power can sometimes seem a daunting affair. The advent of multifocal lens implants and greater patient expectations creates a greater demand for accuracy in predicting the postoperative refractive error. I will attempt to make some of the complexities easier to comprehend by breaking this subject down into its component parts. The three major points of concern are biometry, formulas, and clinical. I will divide biometry into three parts: the axial length, the corneal power and the IOL position. The subject of formulas will be divided into formula generations, formula usage and formula personalization. The clinical area will be segmented into patient needs and desires, special circumstances and problems and errors. Each of these areas will be discussed in depth.

BIOMETRY

Axial Length

If the natural crystalline lens (cataract) is to be removed, obtaining an accurate axial length is mandatory. If the lens has already been removed (aphakia/pseudophakia) or will not be removed (phakic refractive lens), an axial length is not always necessary because the correct implant lens power can be calculated using a refractive formula. Because this formula requires an accurate vertex distance, it is not dependable in cases of aphakia, in which errors in the vertex distance of a high-powered refraction can have a significant effect (Table 4-1).

Table 4-1

Requirements for Obtaining Accurate Axial Length Measurements (in Order of Importance)

- A-scan Ultrasound Instrument
- Real-Time Oscilloscope Screen
- Immersion Technique
- Appropriate Ultrasound Velocities
- Experienced Technician
- B-scan backup

Axial Length Instruments

Until now, all axial length measuring instruments have been A-scan ultrasound units. There are many A-scan instruments available and it is important to make sure the unit that you are using has been calibrated and is capable of accurate measurements. It is important to be sure that the instrument has an oscilloscope screen so that true echo spikes are observed in determining axiality. Instruments that merely report a numerical reading of the axial length ("black box" or spike simulation) do not allow for clinical decision making during the examination and are fraught with potential errors. A major step in improving accuracy would be to replace such an instrument with one that has an oscilloscope screen.

A new methodology for axial length has been introduced by Zeiss/Jena/Humphrey. It is called laser tomography. The instrument is called the IOLMaster and performs four functions; it measures the axial length, the corneal power, the anterior chamber depth, and performs the formula IOL power calculations using modern formulas. We are now performing side-by-side analysis of the accuracy of the instrument compared to standard techniques. Initial reports from Germany (Wolfgang Haigis, PhD) conclude that it cannot obtain results in 10% of eyes because of either density of the cataract or the patient's inability to fixate. Ultrasound will always be needed.

Immersion Technique

The immersion technique of Ossoinig[1] has been shown to be more accurate than the standard applanation technique by many studies[2,3] over the past 25 years. These reports demonstrate a mean average shortening of the axial length of 0.25 to 0.33 mm using applanation compared to immersion. If this error was consistent for all eyes, it could be compensated for by the mere addition of a constant or by personalization. This is not possible because the error varies from eye to eye.

Arguments against immersion are that it is time-consuming, expensive, messy, and requires the patient to be supine. On the contrary, the examination can be performed in a standard ophthalmic examination chair reclined back at a 45 degree angle with the headrest set back so that the patient's axial length is perpendicular to the floor. To maintain a non-leaking fluid bath in the Ossoinig scleral shell, we use a 50/50 dilution of four 15 cc bottles of 2.5% hydroxypropyl methylcellulose 2.5%, (Goniosol) (CIBA Vision

Ophthalmics, Atlanta, Ga) into one 118 cc bottle of Dacriose solution (CIBA Vision Ophthalmics). This is more economical and works well. Once the eye is anesthetized topically, the scleral shell is gently placed between the lids and filled three quarters full with the solution. Any air bubbles should be removed with a short silicone tube attached to a syringe. The latter can also be used to remove the solution at the completion of the procedure. The ultrasound probe is placed into the solution and positioned parallel to the axis of the eye. Axiality is judged by watching for the correct spike patterns on the oscilloscope screen as the probe position is adjusted.

Note: If the axial length is very difficult to obtain and the eye appears to have a length greater than 25 mm, suspect a staphyloma. By direct ophthalmoscopy (with patient fixating on cross hair target), measure the distance from the target (macula) to the optic nerve (in disc diameters). B-scan exam is then performed to measure the axial length at that distance from the edge of the optic nerve shadow.

Note: When measuring an eye containing an IOL, ignore multiple reduplication echoes noted in the vitreous space, which are caused by the IOL.

Note: Anyone planning silicone oil injection into the vitreous space should perform an accurate axial length measurement before doing so and make this information available to the patient.

Try using a sound velocity of 1000 m/sec, but it is practically impossible to measure a silicone oil eye. Alternatively, consider performing a secondary implant after an aphakic refraction is obtained.

Note: Measuring the axial length of both eyes is prudent and customary.

Photographic documentation of the axial length reading is useful and available on many units. Always measure axial length to the nearest hundredth of a millimeter and record it carefully. Errors in axial length are the most significant and amount to approximately 2.5 diopter/mm in IOL power, but it is important to be aware that it drops to approximately 1.75 D/mm in very long eyes (30 mm) and jumps to approximately 3.75 D/mm in very short eyes (20 mm). Greater care must be taken in these short eyes.

Ultrasound Velocities

The ultrasound velocities[4,5] at body temperature for the various parts of the eye and intraocular lens materials have been accepted as:

- Cornea and lens   1641 m/sec
- Aqueous and vitreous   1532 m/sec
- PMMA IOL   2660 m/sec
- Silicone IOL   980 m/sec
- Acrylic IOL   2026 m/sec
- Glass IOL   6040 m/sec
- Silicone oil   987 m/sec

From these values, I calculated average sound speeds[4] for various conditions of a 23.5 mm eye:

- Phakic eye   1555 m/sec
- Aphakic eye   1534 m/sec
- PMMA pseudophakic   1556 m/sec
- Silicone pseudophakic   1476 m/sec
- Acrylic pseudophakic   1549 m/sec
- Glass pseudophakic   1549 m/sec

- Phakic silicone oil   1139 m/sec
- Aphakic silicone oil   1052 m/sec

Note: Measuring an eye containing a silicone IOL with standard phakic velocity (1555 m/sec) can amount to an error of 3 to 4 D.

Because of the inversely proportional change in the axial ratio of solid to liquid as the eye increases in length, the average phakic velocity of a short 20 mm eye is 1560 m/sec, and that of a long 30 mm eye is 1550 m/sec instead of the nominal 1555 m/sec. This factor amounts to only a small (0.25 D) error in the extremes of axial length, but it can be corrected for. This inversely proportional relationship is greater in pseudophakic eyes but is not a factor in aphakic eyes.

If an eye has been measured using the wrong velocity, it can be easily corrected without remeasuring the eye by using the following formula:

AL CORRECTED = (AL MEASURED) x (V CORRECT)/V MEASURED

This is because the instrument does not measure length (D). Instead it measures the time (T) it takes the sound to traverse the eye and converts it to a linear value using the velocity (V) formula where D = VT.

Optional CALF Method

Holladay[6] has offered an optional method to measure the axial length that eliminates the error inherent in changes in average velocity due to the length of the eye. All eyes, regardless of status, are measured at a velocity of 1532 m/sec and to this value is added the corrected axial length factor (CALF). The CALF value represents the thickness of a lens in the eye whether it is a crystalline lens or an IOL. The formula for the CALF of any lens (including the cornea) is CALF = TL (1-1532/VL), where TL = the axial thickness of the lens and VL = the sound velocity through the lens.

Holladay computes the thickness of the human cataractous lens using TL = 4 + age/100, and the sound velocity through the cataract using VL = 1659 - ([age - 10]/2).

Substituting these two formulas into the CALF formula for the crystalline lens yields:

CALF = [4 + age/100] x [1 - 1532/(1659 - [age - 10/2])].

The CALF for the cataractous lens is therefore calculated using only the age of the patient. Holladay recommends using a CALF value of 0.28 (value for 70-year-old) for all ages because the value for a 1-year-old is 0.306 and for a 100-year-old is 0.224. The maximum error in CALF for those younger than 70 is 0.026 (0.07 D), and for those older than 70 is 0.056 (0.14 D). This is within an acceptable range.

The reasoning behind this method is that if an "average" velocity is incorrect, it affects the entire axial length measurement. However, if the estimate of the CALF value is wrong, it only affects a small percentage of the overall axial length (ie, only the lens portion).

This formulation, however, ignores the factor of the corneal thickness (0.55 mm). To correct this, I recommend either:

1. Measure the eye at the aphakic velocity of 1534 m/sec and add CALF of 0.28.
2. Measure with the 1532 m/sec velocity and add CALF of 0.32 (0.28 + 0.037).

A similar method can be used for pseudophakic eyes. Using CALF = TL (1-1532/VL) and the known VL for each IOL material we obtain:

- CALF PMMA = TL (1-1532/2660) = +0.424 x TL
- CALF Silicone = TL (1-1532/980) = -0.563 x TL
- CALF Acrylic = TL (1-1532/2026) = +0.243 TL

The correction for the cornea is calculated the same way:

CALF Cornea = TC (1-1532/1641) = 0.55 (0.066423) = 0.036533 or 0.037

Therefore, knowing the thickness of the implanted IOL, the following formulas can be used:

- PMMA eye AL = AL 1532 + 0.424 TL + 0.037
- Silicone eye AL = AL 1532 - 0.563 TL + 0.037
- Acrylic eye AL = AL 1532 + 0.243 TL + 0.037

The IOL thickness can be obtained from the manufacturer of the IOL if the manufacturer, model number, and dioptric power of the IOL is known. If this is unavailable, Holladay[7] provides a table to use in such situations.

The axial length of an eye containing two IOLs of different materials can be obtained using the following formula:

AL = AL 1532 + T1 (1-1532/V1) + T2 (1-1532/V2) + 0.037

Where T1 and V1 are the thickness and velocity of one IOL and T2 and V2 are the thickness and velocity of the other.

Retinal Thickness Factor

Many formula writers add a specific value to the ultrasonic axial length measurement to take into account the additional distance from the surface of the retina to the level of the receptive end of the cone cells. This value has been estimated to be 0.20 to 0.25 mm and is automatically added to the axial length in some formulas (Binkhorst, Holladay) and not used at all in others (Colenbrander, Hoffer Q). Since the Zeiss IOLMaster measures to the cones, a retinal thickness factor (RTF) should not be added.

Corneal Power

The important factors to consider in obtaining accurate corneal power are:

- Instrumentation
- Contact lens wear
- Astigmatism
- Previous refractive surgery
- Corneal transplant eyes

Instrumentation

The corneal power is usually measured by a manual keratometer that measures the front surface of the cornea and converts the radius (r) of curvature obtained to diopters (K) using an index of refraction (IR) of 1.3375 (K = 337.5/r). Many postulate that this index is too high and Holladay[6] recommends using 4/3 instead. To correct for this, multiply the K reading obtained by the factor 0.98765431, which will result in a 0.54 D decrease in corneal power (range 0.43 D for 35 D cornea to 0.62 D for 50 D cornea). If your keratometer uses a different IR, use 1/3/(IR-1) instead.

Note: Before using this refractive index correction factor clinically, test it out on a series of previously operated eyes to see what effect it would have had on your accuracy.

To assure accuracy, it is important to calibrate the keratometer on a regular schedule.

Corneal topography units also supply corneal power values. I performed a prospective comparison study of the manual keratometer (Bausch & Lomb, Claremont, Calif) with one such unit (TechnoMed C-Scan, Tubinger, Germany) on 172 cataract eyes. The mean of the central (3 mm zone) readings was 0.24 D flatter with the topography unit (43.55 D vs. 43.79 D), which may be explained by the index of refraction discussed above. When personalization was performed on both instrument data sets, however, IOL power calculation accuracy was statistically equal.

Note: Hard contact lenses should be removed permanently for at least 2 weeks prior to measuring corneal power for IOL power calculation.

Astigmatism

Regular astigmatism is not a factor in IOL power calculation because the goal is to predict the postoperative spherical equivalent refractive error. Therefore, the average of the two K readings is the only value used, which should result in mixed astigmatism. If a myopic cylinder is desired, the flattest K reading could be used instead. If astigmatism is surgically corrected at the time of lens implantation, it would be important to know the effect of this surgery on the final average corneal power and to adjust the K reading used to calculate the IOL power. Due to the coupling ratio, this effect is usually zero, but an analysis of your previous cases would be useful.

I noted a 0.17 D increase in spherical equivalent of the cornea 1 year after 2.5 mm clear corneal oblique surgery, which should be added to my preoperative/operative K reading.

Previous Refractive Surgery

Previous corneal refractive surgery changes the architecture of the cornea so that standard methods of measuring the corneal power cause it to be overestimated. Radial keratotomy (RK) causes a relatively proportional equal flattening of both the front and back surface of the cornea, which leaves the index of refraction relationship the same. On the other hand, photorefractive keratectomy (PRK) and laser-assisted in-situ keratomileusis (LASIK) flatten only the front surface. This changes the refractive index calculation, creating an overestimation of the corneal power by about 1 D for every 7 D of refractive surgery correction obtained.

The major cause of error is the fact that manual keratometers measure at the 3.2 mm zone of the central cornea, which often misses the central flatter zone of effective corneal power. There are two methods to better estimate the corneal power in these refractive surgery eyes.

Clinical History Method

This method[8-14] is based on the fact that the final change in refractive error the eye obtains from surgery was due only to a change in the effective corneal power. If this change (at the corneal plane) is added to the presurgical corneal power, we will obtain the present effective corneal power.

Note: All patients having corneal refractive surgery should be given the following data to maintain in their personal health records. They should be told to give it to anyone planning to perform cataract/IOL surgery on them.
- Preoperative corneal power
- Preoperative refractive error (spectacle with vertex distance or contact lens power)
- Postoperative healed refractive error (before lens changes affected it)

All attempts should be made to obtain the above information from the refractive surgeon's records. Each spherical equivalent refractive error (R) should be vertex (v) corrected to the corneal plane (0 mm) using: $R_0 = R_v/(1 - V \times R_v)$, or using vertex of 12 mm: $R_0 = R_{12}/1 - 0.012R_{12}$.

The estimated effective corneal power (K) can be calculated using the following formula: $K = K_{PREOP} + R_{PREOP_0} - R_{PO_0}$

Contact Lens Method

This method[8-14] is based on the principle that if a hard contact lens (CL) of plano power (P) and a base curve (B) equal to the effective power of the cornea is placed on the eye, it will not change the refractive error of the eye. That is, the difference between the manifest refraction with the contact lens (R_{CL}) and without it (R_{NoCL}) is zero. The formula to calculate the estimated corneal power is: $K = B + P + R_{CL} - R_{NoCL}$.

The refractive errors should also be vertex-corrected. Several computer IOL power calculation programs calculate these two methods automatically when needed. If the results of both methods are different, use the lowest estimated corneal power. Rarely are such eyes myopic after IOL surgery.

Obviously, the former method cannot be used if the historical data is not available, and the latter is impossible if the cataract precludes performing a refraction. In such cases, it might be wise to delay the IOL implantation and calculate the secondary implant power using the aphakic refractive error in the refraction formula or use a piggyback lens or PRL to correct any deficiency.

Some have recommended fooling the IOL power formula by using the preoperative corneal power and requesting the postoperative refractive error to be what it was prior to refractive surgery.

Corneal Transplant Eyes

A problem also arises when attempting to predict what the corneal power will be after a corneal transplant. Some have suggested using the corneal power of the other eye (if it is available) or using an average of one's post-transplant corneal powers. Published reports, however, show a very large range of prediction and refractive errors using these attempts. Performing the IOL implantation after the corneal transplant has stabilized was suggested by the author[15,16] in 1986. In 1990, Geggle[17] reported excellent refractive results using this two-stepped approach (66% 20/40 or better acuity without correction). A secondary piggyback IOL or PRL is another alternative to correct residual ametropia.

IOL Position

This factor was historically referred to as the anterior chamber depth (ACD) because the optic of all IOLs in the early era was positioned in front of the iris. Because most IOLs today are behind the iris, new terminology has been offered, such as effective lens position (ELP) by Holladay[6] and actual lens position (ALP) by the US Food and Drug Administration (FDA).

IOL position is defined as the axial distance between the two lenses (cornea and IOL), or more exactly, the distance from the front surface (vertex) of the cornea to the effective principle plane of the IOL. This value is required for all formulas and is incorporated into the A constant specific to each IOL style for regression formulas or as an ACD, both of which are supplied by the manufacturer. Some have proposed that it would be useful to measure the preoperative anatomic ACD (corneal epithelium to anterior capsule) either with an A-scan unit or by optical pachymetry. A comparison study we performed on 44 eyes showed that the optical method resulted in a mean 0.20 (±0.35) mm deeper ACD than obtained by ultrasound using 1548 m/sec (3.14 vs 2.93 mm).

The IOL position has been considered the least important of the three variables as a cause of IOL power error, but in 1998 I saw a patient with a shallowed ACD and myopia of −2.50 go to plano in 3 days after the chamber deepened by 2.0 mm. IOL position has received the most attention from formula writers over the past 10 years. The major effort has been toward better prediction of where the IOL will ultimately rest. A recent study I performed on a series of 270 eyes receiving a silicone plate haptic lens showed that the IOL shifted a mean of 0.06 mm posteriorly at 3 months compared to its position on the first day after surgery. This was commensurate with a mean 0.21 D shift toward hyperopia. It could be postulated that it should have shifted anteriorly as the capsule tightened up.

FORMULAS

Generations

First Generation

The first IOL power formula was published by Fyodorov[18] in 1967. Colenbrander[19] wrote his in 1972, followed by the Hoffer[20] formula in 1974. Binkhorst[21] published his formula in 1975, which became widely used in America. In 1978, Lloyd and Gills,[22,23] followed by Retzlaff[24] and later Sanders and Kraff[25], each developed a regression formula based on analysis of their previous IOL cases. This work was amalgamated in 1980 to yield the SRK I formula.[26] All these formulas depended on a single constant for each lens that represented the predicted IOL position (ACD).

Second Generation

In 1980, at the Welsh Cataract Congress in Houston, I showed a direct relationship between the position of a PMMA posterior chamber IOL and the axial length and presented a formula to better predict ACD[27,28]. Others (Binkhorst,[29] SRK II[30]) developed different mechanisms to apply this predictive relationship, which Holladay defined as the second generation.

Third Generation

In 1988, Holladay[31] proposed a direct relationship between the steepness of the cornea and the position of the IOL. He modified the Binkhorst formula to incorporate this, as well as the axial length relationship. Instead of ACD input, the formula would calculate the predicted distance from the cornea to the iris plane and add to it the distance from the iris plane to the IOL. The latter he called the surgeon factor (SF), and it is specific to each lens. Retzlaff[32] followed suit and modified the Holladay I formula to allow use of A constants, calling it the SRK/T theoretic formula in 1990. It was intended to replace the previous SRK regression formulas, but still 50% of American surgeons use them. In 1992, Hoffer developed the Q formula[33] to accomplish the same effect.

Fourth Generation

In 1990, Olsen[34] proposed using the preoperative ACD and other factors to better estimate the postoperative IOL position, and published algorithms for this. After several studies showed that the Holladay I formula was not as accurate as the Hoffer Q in eyes shorter than 22 mm, Holladay used the preoperative ACD measurement as well as corneal diameter, lens thickness, refractive error, and age to calculate an estimated scaling factor (ESF) that adjusts the IOL-specific ACD. This Holladay 2 formula has been promulgated since 1996 but has yet to be published.

Refraction Formula

Holladay[35] published a formula in 1993 to calculate the power of an IOL for an aphakic eye or ametropic pseudophakic eye (piggyback IOL), or a phakic refractive lens (PRL) for a phakic eye. It does not need the axial length but requires the corneal power, preoperative refractive error, and desired postoperative refractive error as well as the vertex distance of both. I do not recommend its use in aphakic eyes because the vertex distance is difficult to measure accurately, and due to the high power of their refractive error, greater errors can result. It is, however, a good check against the axial length formula calculation.

Usage

Based on Axial length

My study[33] showed that in the normal range (72%) of axial length (22.0 to24.5 mm), almost all formulas function adequately, but the SRK I formula is the leading cause of poor refractive results in eyes outside this range. It also showed that the Holladay I formula was the most accurate in medium long eyes (24.5 to 26.0 mm) (15%) and the SRK/T was more accurate in very long eyes (>26.0 mm) (5%). In short eyes (<22.0 mm) (8%), the Hoffer Q formula was the most accurate; this was confirmed in an additional large study of 830 short eyes (p>0.0001) as well as in a multiple-surgeon study by Holladay. A more recent study[42] that I performed of 317 eyes showed that the Holladay 2 formula equaled the Hoffer Q in short eyes but was not as accurate as the Holladay I or Hoffer Q in average and medium long eyes. Eyes shorter than 19 mm are extremely rare (0.1 %) and may well be helped by using the Holladay 2 formula. Holladay has postulated that the other formulas overestimate the shallowing of the effective lens position (ELP) in these very short eyes.

Methodology

There are several means by which to use these newer formulas, including A-scans, hand-held calculators, and computer programs that run on DOS, Windows, Macintosh, and Palm operating systems. You can also program the published formulas on a spreadsheet program. The most popular commercial programs are the Hoffer Programs System (1994) and the Holladay IOL Consultant (1997) (Eye Lab Inc., Santa Monica, Calif.), which include several formulas and the ability to personalize them, as well as routines to deal with odd clinical situations such as radial keratotomy (RK) eyes and piggyback IOLs.

Personalization

The concept of personalizing a formula based on a surgeon's past experience and data was introduced by Retzlaff[36] using the A constant to refine the formula. Holladay incorporated this concept into backsolving for the surgeon factor, and Hoffer backsolved for his personalized ACD. Several studies have proved that formula personalization definitely significantly improves formula accuracy.

The following parameters are required from postoperative eyes:
- Axial length (preoperative)
- Corneal power (preoperative)
- IOL power
- Postoperative refractive error (stable)

The eyes should all contain the same lens style by the same manufacturer implanted by the same surgeon. The same biometry instruments and technician should also have been used. Eyes with postoperative surprises or acuity worse than 20/40 should not be included due to poor accuracy in obtaining refractive error.

CLINICAL

Patient Needs and Desires

Most surgeons have developed their own plan for deciding on the clinical needs of their patients. When implanting monofocal IOLs, it has often been recommended to aim patients for mild postoperative myopia (-0.5 to -1.5 D) so that if the error is on the plus side, they will be emmetropic; and if on the minus side, they will have reading vision. This is necessary because of the larger range of IOL power errors generally experienced. When the bell-shaped curve of prediction error is squeezed down to 67% within ±0.50 D, it is then possible to aim most patients for emmetropia. This is even more important when implanting a multifocal IOL. Senior citizens are much more active today than in the past, and in emergency situations it would be much safer if they were emmetropic rather than looking around for their myopic correction to escape to safety.

There are several exceptions, however. Patients who have been long-term myopes are never happy being hyperopes postoperatively. Patients that would wind up with a large anisometropia should be stimulated to be fit with a contact lens in the other eye prior to deciding on an emmetropic IOL. Monocular CL wearers are more successful than binocular. It is wise to document all discussions in unusual situations.

Special Circumstances

Monocular Cataract in Bilateral Large Ametropia

The dilemma is to make the surgical eye emmetropic or to match the large ametropia of the other eye, which may never need surgery. Until now, I have convinced patients to accept a CL or ignore the other eye and go for the "brass ring" of emmetropia. In the future, those that cannot tolerate CLs could have a PRL placed over the IOL to eliminate aneisikonia and have it removed if the other eye ultimately has surgery. Or, the highly myopic eye could be corrected with a phakic refractive lens (PRL).

Pediatric Eyes

Children have always posed a dilemma[37] in IOL power selection in that the eye will grow in length and become more myopic if a fixed emmetropic power is implanted. The study of pediatric eyes by Gordon and Donzis[38] shows a steep axial length growth rate from premature babies to age 2 increasing by 6 mm (approximately 20 D), while corneal power drops from 54 D to 44 D, offsetting 10 D. If IOLs are used in this age group, it might be best to place piggyback lenses with the more posterior IOL, having the average adult emmetropic power and the anterior IOL being the added power needed to reach emmetropia now. As the child grows, he or she can be corrected with myopic glasses until he or she is old enough to have the anterior IOL removed.

Between the ages of 2 to 5 years, growth slows to about 0.4 mm per year and only increases another 1 mm from age 5 to 10 while corneal power remains stable. From age 2 to 10, it might be wise to aim for 1.5 to 2 D of hyperopia postoperatively, which allows for reasonable uncorrected vision and light spectacle correction in amblyopia treatment. When the child matures, he or she will wind up emmetropic or mildly myopic, depending on age at implantation. Growth slows after age 10 to 15, and emmetropia can be the aim. Future use of implantable PRL over the top of IOLs may be very helpful in these children since they can easily be exchanged as the eye grows, keeping the child emmetropic throughout life.

Bifocal IOL

In 1991,[39] I reported that to obtain -2.75 D myopia (reading at 14 to 16 inches) the IOL must be about 3.75 to 4.00 D stronger than the emmetropic power. I also showed that the amount of this additional power in a bifocal IOL is not affected by the axial length and very little by the corneal power. It is affected, however, by the IOL position and an anterior chamber (AC) lens would need less add power than a posterior chamber (PC) lens. Obviously, to negate the need for any glasses, it is important to aim for emmetropia, but mild postoperative hyperopia is far better than even the mildest myopia. The distance vision will be reasonable in the former (they can easily obtain readers if necessary), while in the latter it will not. Bifocal IOL patients with myopia are not happy, and everything should be done to avoid this situation since minus power "readers" are not readily available. In the future, a PRL could be implanted over the top of the bifocal to make the eye emmetropic.

Silicone Oil Refractive Effect

The second problem that arises when the vitreous is replaced with silicone oil is that the refractive index of the oil is much less than that of vitreous, and it acts as a negative lens in the eye, which must be offset with more power in the IOL. This effect is dependent upon the shape factor of the back surface of the IOL such that a biconvex IOL creates the worst problem and a concave posterior lens causes practically none. In between the two is the plano-posterior lens, which is recommended in these cases. With a plano-convex lens, 2 to 3 D must be added to the IOL power to compensate for this issue.

Piggyback Lenses

Piggyback lenses can either be placed primarily, or the second lens placed secondarily, over a previously healed IOL. In the former, the anterior IOL forces the posterior IOL

more posteriorly a distance equal to the central thickness of the anterior lens. This causes the posterior lens (whose focal point is moved farther behind the retina) to require
more power to maintain the same focus. This effect is lessened by a thinner (lower
power) anterior lens, and a thinner lens is easier to remove if necessary. Primary piggyback lenses need special calculations to adjust for the posterior lens shift.

Secondary lenses can be calculated using the refraction formula or by a more simple
formulation based on the fact that the healed primary IOL is more stable. Due to the different effect on vertex power changes between plus and minus lenses, the following formulation works well.

Piggyback IOL = 1.5 x Rx Hyperopic or = 1.0 x Rx Myopic

Problems and Errors

The major problem is an unacceptable postoperative refractive error. The sooner it is
discovered, the sooner it can be corrected and the patient made happy. Therefore, it is
wise to perform K readings and refraction on the first postoperative day. Immediate surgical correction[40] (24 to 48 hours) will allow easy access to the incision and the capsular
bag, will create only one postoperative period, and will result in excellent uncorrected
vision. Until now, we could only correct this by lens exchange, which creates the dilemma of determining which factor created the IOL power error: axial length, corneal power,
or mislabeled IOL. Today, with the advent of low-powered IOLs, the best remedy is a piggyback IOL. It is not necessary to determine what caused the error or to remeasure the
axial length of the freshly operated pseudophakic eye.

It is important to remember that a shallow AC can lead to as much as 3 D of myopia
(depending on the power of the IOL), which will disappear when the AC reforms. An RK
eye has a propensity for the cornea to flatten postoperatively, causing large hyperopic
surprises. It may take up to 3 or 4 months for the cornea to resteepen; therefore, surgical correction should not be attempted until then.

CONCLUSION

Simple steps and attention to detail can be very useful in preventing IOL power errors,
but recent advances in IOL power range availability have made this problem more easily corrected. This is an ever-changing science and new developments are sure to come.

REFERENCES

1. Ossoinig KC. Standardized echography: basic principles, clinical applications, and results. *Int Ophthalmol Clin*. 1979;19(4):127.

2. Shammas HJF. A comparison of immersion and contact techniques for axial length meas-
    urements. *Am Intraocular Implant Soc J*. 1984;10:444-447.

3. Schelenz J, Kammann J. Comparison of contact and immersion techniques for axial meas-
    urement and implant power calculation. *J Cataract Refract Surg*. 1989;15:425-428.

4. Hoffer KJ. Ultrasound speeds for axial length measurement. *J Cataract Refract Surg*. 1994;
    20:554-562.

5. *Encyclopedia of Polymer Science and Engineering*. Vol 1. New York: Wiley and Sons;
    1989;147-149.

6. Holladay JT. Standardizing constants for ultrasonic biometry, keratometry, and intraocular
    lens power calculation. *J Cataract Refract Surg*. 1997;23:1356-1370.

7. Holladay JT, Prager TC. Accurate ultrasonic biometry in pseudophakia. *Amer J Ophthalmol.* 1989;107:189-190.

8. Holladay JT. IOL calculations following radial keratotomy surgery. *Refract Corneal Surg.* 1989;5:36A.

9. Hoffer KJ. IOL power calculation in RK eyes. *Phaco & Foldables.* 1994;7(3):6.

10. Hoffer KJ. Calculation of intraocular lens power in post-radial keratotomy eyes. *Ophthalmic Practice* (Canada). 1994;12(5):242-243.

11. Hoffer KJ. Ways to calculate IOL power in RK eyes. Refractive surgery update (Thornton). *Ocular Surg News.* 1995;13(10):86.

12. Hoffer KJ. Intraocular lens power calculation for eyes after refractive keratotomy. *J Refract Surg.* 1995;11:490-493.

13. Hoffer KJ. How to do cataract surgery after RK. *Review of Ophthalmol.* 1996;20:117-120.

14. Hoffer KJ. Intraocular lens power calculation for eyes after refractive keratotomy. Consultation Section. *Ann Ophthalmol.* 1996;28(2):67-68.

15. Hoffer KJ. The triple procedure: a plea for three. *Geriatric Ophthalmol.* 1986;2(3):7.

16. Hoffer KJ. Triple procedure for intraocular lens exchange. *Arch Ophthalmol.* 1987;105:609.

17. Geggel HS. Intraocular lens implantation after penetrating keratoplasty: improved unaided visual acuity, astigmatism, and safety in patients with combined corneal disease and cataract. *Ophthalmol.* 1990;97:1460-1467.

18. Fyodorov SN, Kolonko AI. Estimation of optical power of the intraocular lens. *Vestnik Oftalmologic* (Moscow). 1967;4:27.

19. Colenbrander MC. Calculation of the power of an iris-clip lens for distance vision. *Brit J Ophthalmol.* 1973;57:735-740.

20. Hoffer KJ. Intraocular lens calculation: the problem of the short eye. *Ophthalmic Surg.* 1981;12:269-272.

21. Binkhorst RD. The optical design of intraocular lens implants. *Ophthalmic Surg.* 1975;6(3):17-31.

22. Gills JP. Regression formula (editorial). *Am Intra-Ocular Implant Soc J.* 1978;4:163.

23. Gills JP. Minimizing postoperative refractive error. *Contact and Intraocular Lens Med J.* 1980;6:56-59.

24. Retzlaff J. A new intraocular lens calculation formula. *Am Intra-Ocular Implant Soc J.* 1980;6:148.

25. Sanders DR, Kraff MC. Improvement of intraocular lens power calculation: regression formula. *Am Intra-Ocular Implant Soc J.* 1980; 6:263.

26. Sanders DR, Retzlaff J, Kraff MC, et al. Comparison of the accuracy of the Binkhorst, Colenbrander and SRK implant power prediction formulas. *Am Intra-Ocular Implant Soc J.* 1981;7:337-340.

27. Hoffer KJ. Biometry of the posterior capsule: A new formula for anterior chamber depth of posterior chamber lenses. In: Emery JC, Jacobson AC, Eds. *Current Concepts in Cataract Surgery* (Eighth Congress). New York: Appleton-Century Crofts. 1983;56-62.

28. Hoffer KJ. The effect of axial length on posterior chamber lenses and posterior capsule position. *Current Concepts in Ophthalmic Surg.* 1984;1:20-22.

29. Binkhorst RD. Biometric A-scan ultrasonography and intraocular lens power calculation. In: Emery JE, ed. *Current Concepts in Cataract Surgery: Selected Proceedings of the Fifth Biennial Cataract Surgical Congress.* St. Louis, Mo: Mosby CV; 1987:175-182.

30. Sanders DR, Retzlaff J, Kraff MC. Comparison of the SRK II formula and the other second generation formulas. *J Cataract Refract Surg.* 1988;14:136-141.

31. Holladay JT, Prager TC, Chandler TY, Musgrove KH. A three-part system for refining intraocular lens power calculations. *J Cataract Refract Surg.* 1988;14:17-24.

32. Retzlaff J, Sanders DR, Kraff MC. Development of the SRK/T intraocular lens implant power calculation formula. *J Cataract Refract Surg.* 1990;16:333-340.

33. Hoffer KJ. The Hoffer Q formula: a comparison of theoretic and regression formulas. *J Cataract Refract Surg.* 1993;19:700-712. Errata: 1994;20:677.

34. Olsen T, Oleson H, Thim K, Corydon L. Prediction of postoperative intraocular lens chamber depth. *J Cataract Refract Surg.* 1990; 16:587-590.

35. Holladay JT. Refractive power calculation for intraocular lenses in the phakic eye. *Amer J Ophthalmol.* 1993;116:63-66.

36. Retzlaff J. Calculating the surgeon's personal A-constant. In: Retzlaff J, Sanders DR, Kraff MC, eds. *Lens Implant Power Calculation Manual.* 3rd ed. Thorofare, NJ: SLACK Incorporated;1990:12-13.

37. Hoffer KJ. Selection of lens power for implantation in infants and children. *Am Intra-Ocular Implant Soc J.* 1975;1(2):49.

38. Gordon RA, Donzis PB. Refractive development of the human eye. *Arch Ophthalmol.* 1985;103:785-789.

39. Hoffer KJ. Lens power calculation for multifocal IOLs. In: Maxwell A, Nordan, LT, eds. *Current Concepts of Multifocal Intraocular Lenses.* Thorofare, NJ: SLACK Incorporated:1991;193-208.

40. Hoffer KJ. Early lens exchange for power calculation error. *J Cataract Refract Surg.* 1995;21: 486-487.

41. Hoffer KJ. Modern IOL power calculations: avoiding errors and planning for special circumstances. *Focal Points, American Academy of Ophthalmology.* 1999;XVII(12):1-9.

42. Hoffer KJ. Clinical results using the Holladay 2 IOL power formula. *J Cataract Refract Surg.* 2000;In press.

5 Outcomes Analysis for IOL Calculations

R. Bruce Wallace III, MD

THE BENEFITS OF OUTCOMES ANALYSIS

Outcomes analysis has been a mainstay in clinical trials for medical devices, such as the Array multifocal IOL, for many years. After reporting the results of improvements in visual acuity and visual function with the Array lens, the US Food and Drug Administration (FDA) was satisfied that this technology could be an effective method to provide uncorrected multifocal vision after cataract surgery. What is often overlooked, however, is that outcomes analysis can be a valuable tool within our surgical practices.

The benefits of measuring the outcome of a given procedure are two-fold. First, we can judge the effectiveness and improvement our treatment has provided for our patients. Second, and more important, by continuing to follow our results, we stimulate a keen desire to steadily improve. Unfortunately, outcomes analysis is not easy. Even though new tools are now available to help in this area, such as computer software, measuring outcomes requires a time commitment by knowledgeable staff in order to assemble reliable data. When offices embark on this new journey into data collection, frustration and skepticism commonly emerge. There never appears to be enough time for this task to be performed. One reason for this initial negative attitude is that the fruits of the efforts come later, after demonstrating improvements in results. To help convince cataract surgeons of the benefits of surgical outcomes analysis, I like to use a familiar data collection effort used by many medical practices, that of "wait time studies."

Intermittently, medical practices assess how long patients are kept waiting in the reception area before a routine clinic exam. Wait time studies are a helpful barometer of office efficiency. When we have engaged in these studies, I have found that my office staff seems to work smarter and faster than usual. Why is this? One reason is that the technicians know they are being evaluated for their ability to see patients on time. Simply by knowing that they are being rated for a given task, they tend to improve their performance of this task, almost subconsciously. Imagine how much effort an athlete would put forth if nobody kept score. We have learned that outcomes analysis by itself creates an incentive for improving results.

Outcomes analysis can be viewed as a four-step process. By using these four steps, our office team has seen significant improvements in IOL power calculations, and recently, in reducing astigmatism during cataract surgery. Accurate IOL power calculations and minimal postoperative astigmatism are key ingredients for refractive cataract surgery, especially for multifocal IOL implantation. Let's review these four steps of outcomes analysis in general terms.

THE FOUR STEPS OF OUTCOMES ANALYSIS

Setting Goals for Improvement

Setting goals requires the team to have specific knowledge of how effective and accurate they already are with whatever they are trying to improve. Therefore, an initial assessment is needed. Then the team sets specific goals for improvement over a given period of time. Everyone on the team needs to understand the importance of reaching these goals, and their responsibilities in the improvement process. Ideally, the entire team should be convinced that these goals are valuable and attainable.

Uncovering Sources of Error

Once the team knows where it is and where it wants to be, the only way to improve performance is to remove or reduce as many flaws as possible from the system. System analysis (that is, carefully examining each step in a given area of patient care to look for errors) gives the team clues as to the changes in the system that can lead to better results. A common example of error in IOL calculations is neglecting to personalize lens constants. However, once the office team identifies this flaw as an obstacle to reaching its goal for improvement in IOL accuracy, a commitment to adding personalization of lens constants is more likely to take place.

Improving Techniques

The various impediments to improvement have now been identified and the team moves forward toward its goals. Better techniques sometimes involve better equipment, more training, and sometimes just better attitudes about the importance of the team pulling together for the common good of the goals set forth. This step involves a commitment to "paying the price." By remaining curious about new methods and keeping an open mind to new ideas, the goals will be easier to obtain. On the other hand, remaining in the comfort zone of the status quo is a common obstacle to improvement and often emerges as a source of error.

Improving Results

Regular assessments of effective team performance will often demonstrate improvement. Better results are the rewards the team enjoys after working together to improve its efforts. The team should celebrate success as it moves on the road to the agreed upon goals. When results are less than anticipated, the team returns to steps two and three in order to move forward again.

The Patient Satisfaction Program

Background

Since 1991, our office has been utilizing monthly outcomes analysis for IOL calculations, which we have termed "The Patient Satisfaction Program" (PSP). As the name implies, the more accurate we are with IOL power calculations, the happier our patients will be with their surgical results. Let's take a look at how PSP was designed. First, we knew that the best accuracy level achievable with present-day ultrasound and keratometry was within ± 0.50 D (that is why IOLs come in half diopter steps). Therefore, we set a spherical equivalent target for each eye, preoperatively hoping to be within ± 0.50 D of that target. We then measured our postoperative spherical equivalent results, usually 1 month after surgery, assuming a stable refraction had been reached. We then determined how often we were within 0.50 D of our intended target. We started with a 47% level of accuracy in 1991, a lower accuracy level than we expected to find. However, by utilizing the four steps of outcomes analysis, we began to witness steady improvement. By March of 1996, our PSP reached 80% accuracy. We have remained in this range since that time.

Data Processing

Computer programs are being developed to help in the task of following IOL calculation accuracy. If one of these programs is not available, random sampling can be used instead. With this method, the team pulls postoperative charts at random with at least a 1-month follow-up. We look for patients with accurate refractions (with good vision of 20/20 or 20/25). When determining IOL calculation accuracy, random sampling can also be employed in personalizing lens constants. Fortunately, many newer computer software programs automatically calculate this information once the postoperative data is entered in the program.

Troubleshooting

Following the four steps of outcomes analysis includes learning from mistakes in the IOL calculation process. Imagine that during random sampling, we encounter an unexpected result, especially hyperopia. Obviously, this represents an unwanted event and signals a possible flaw in the preoperative assessment for the IOL calculation. The team needs to re-analyze the clinical information that was acquired preoperatively and attempt to uncover the source of error. A stepwise assessment would include:

- **Evaluating the A-scan echogram**. Do the spikes appear reliable? Is the anterior chamber depth appropriate for this eye?
- **What was the technician's A-scan rating?** Each technician performing A-scans should rate the reliability of his or her scan based on reproducibility of the axial length and the cooperation of the patient.
- **Was this a new IOL? Was it placed "in the bag"?** The initial experience with another IOL can lead to unexpected refractive results until personalization of the surgeon's lens constant takes place. Rarely, the lens may be in the correct location inside the eye, such as resting in the ciliary sulcus rather than in the capsular bag.

- **Should the A-scan be remeasured?** If the refractive result cannot be explained, consideration should be given to performing another A-scan for this eye postoperatively, especially if surgery is anticipated in the fellow eye.

The Team Approach

As with all outcomes analysis, each member of the team involved with patient care needs to be made aware of the importance of accurate IOL calculations. By naming our efforts the Patient Satisfaction Program, we have sent a clear message to our staff of the value that better uncorrected vision has to our cataract patients. Our results are reported to all of our employees during our staff meetings. By sharing these results, we continue to stimulate a desire for continued improvement.

Outcomes analysis in eye surgery will continue to grow in popularity. Already, there are agencies that plan to publish outcomes of various cataract surgery centers on the Internet. While for many this action appears like an invasion of privacy, a number of these participating practices will be stimulated to improve their results. Along with improved visual acuity (both uncorrected and corrected, distance and near) will be the assessment of improvements in visual function (ie, "quality of life" studies).

Refractive cataract surgeons should be proactive in outcomes analysis, because in the long run our patients are the principal beneficiaries of our efforts to improve our results.

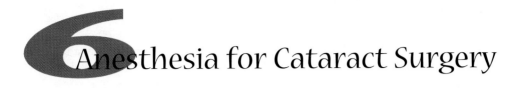

6 Anesthesia for Cataract Surgery

David M. Dillman, MD

INTRODUCTION

Augusta National Golf Club is one of the most exclusive clubs in the world. Membership is by invitation only, and for many years was run by an autocratic chairman, Cliff Roberts, a Wall Street financier who had total control over the place, including the comings and goings on the membership roster. If Roberts decided you were no longer going to be a member, you were history. No letter, no appeal. According to one story, the process went something like this:

A member called the club to arrange for a visit and a stay in one of the cabins. The switchboard connected him with Mr. Roberts, who informed him that he was no longer a member.

"For what reason, Cliff?" the astonished man asked.

"Nonpayment of your bill," said Roberts coldly.

"But, I never received a bill," the member protested.

"Exactly," said Roberts, as he hung up the phone.

No such thing as a free lunch works in cataract surgery as well.

The challenges we face in lens/IOL surgery—to identify and obtain that elusive "state of the art" status—can be staggering. Many are contained in this text. Here's the good news: This chapter is a simple one… straightforward and low tech.

PUPIL DILATION

As President, Jimmy Carter was not known for his sense of humor, but he got off a good one during a visit to Egypt after he was told that the Great Pyramid of Giza took 20 years to build. Said Carter, "I'm surprised that a government organization could do it that quickly." That's the purpose of this section— not to tell you how to dilate a pupil—but how to do it quickly and efficiently. I learned it from some colleagues whom I believe learned it from Jim Gills at the 1999 American Academy of Ophthalmology meeting. However, the real credit for the concept goes to Ken Rosenthal, MD. He developed the basic process in 1992 and presented it at the 1993 American Society of Cataract and Refractive Surgery meeting.

Here are the steps for your preoperative nursing staff to follow:
1. Create a dilating "cocktail." The ingredients of this concoction are basically a mixture of the preoperative drops you currently use. The exact amounts you will determine by trial and error. Here's what we are using at the present time in my practice:
    a. 2.5 cc Cyclogyl 1%
    b. 2.5 cc Neosynephrine 2.5%
    c. 1 cc Ocufen
    d. 1 cc Ciloxan
They are mixed together to give a total of 7 cc of our potion.
2. Soak small cotton balls in the above mixture. We use prerolled dental pledgets (they come in various sizes; we use size #3), but you could make your own. Instead of cotton, you may also cut instrument wipes into small pieces.
3. Upon arrival to the surgery facility, place a drop or two of your favorite topical anesthetic (Tetracaine, Alcaine, Ophthaine, etc.) into the inferior conjunctival fornix.
4. Place a soaked cotton ball into the inferior conjunctival fornix. We try to line it up with the pupil.
5. Then, if I may borrow from the Sopranos, "F'get about it." Just leave it alone and let it do its thing. Give it about 30 minutes and you should have a nicely dilated pupil without the hassle of repeated applications.
6. Once in the operating room, have the person doing the eye/skin prep remove the cotton ball and discard it.

History of Topical Anesthesia

"Some men see things that are and ask why. I dream things that never were and say why not?"

—Robert Kennedy

I don't know exactly who deserves the credit as the absolute first cataract surgeon to use topical anesthesia. I do know of at least two earlier reports that were brought to my attention by Dr. Charles H. Williamson.[1] In 1910, Dr. Julius Hirschberg reported the use of a 2% cocaine solution in thousands of cataract surgeries and "encountered only advantages, never a single disadvantage." Using a combination of topical anesthesia and superior subconjunctival lidocaine injection, Dr. R. Smith of London performed planned extracapsular cataract extraction (ECCE) in 175 cases from 1985 to 1988.[2]

As far as I'm concerned, however, Richard Fichman, MD of Manchester, Conn is solely responsible for bringing topical anesthesia to small incision cataract surgery. His foresight, and his courage to challenge tradition, has had such a wonderfully positive impact upon my ability to deliver (what I consider to be) full impact, state-of-the-art cataract surgery to my patients. In a personal interview, he was willing to share with me the road he traveled in order to reach such a grand destination.

Dr. Fichman's arrival at topical anesthesia was along a path paved with a series of "whys" and "why nots." In early 1991, after performing small-incision, self-sealing cataract surgery, he was struck by the fact that his patients suffered little pain from the cataract surgery itself. However, too many patients experienced pain with the regional block and/or had nausea and malaise from the accompanying intravenous medications. A serendipitous problem with a batch of hyaluronidase (Wydase) started the cascade. It gave him the opportunity to challenge: "Is Wydase really necessary? Why do we use it?

Why not try the block without it?" He stopped incorporating Wydase and observed no intraoperative or postoperative differences.

Next was bupivacaine HCL (Marcaine). Fichman had been taught to use it as a resident when ECCE was the order of the day. "Why do I use it now with my current technique? Is it really necessary? Why not try the block without it?" He stopped incorporating Marcaine and observed only positive differences (quicker return of acuity, lid movement, and ocular movement).

Now, using only lidocaine HCL (Xylocaine), he began to see some of his patients a few hours after surgery (rather than waiting until the following day). Within that time frame, he noted that good visual function was returning and that the patients were happier and much better off without the traditional overnight patch. He was only one step away.

That summer, he took a radial keratotomy course that, ironically, changed the course of cataract surgery. He learned that a Russian-style (uphill) RK incision could be made with topical anesthesia only. In some respects, that struck him as being potentially more troublesome than his tightly controlled small-incision cataract surgery.

Upon his return, he decreased his 5 cc 2% Xylocaine required block to 4 cc. In short order, it went to 3 cc, then 2 cc, then 1 cc. Then came the final "why not."

In September 1991, he performed his first small-incision cataract surgery using only topical tetracaine HCL. Understandably, he performed his first "10 to 15 cases with my heart in my throat." But, to his absolute delight, he found these patients to be positively "different in every aspect." As a group, they were happier and more enthusiastic than any of his previous cataract surgery patients. For the first time in his professional career, he asked his wife to come into the office to see and share the tremendously wonderful impact this phenomenon was having on his patients, his staff, and himself.

Later that year, at a small meeting in Stowe, Vt, he shared, for the first time with some colleagues, his discovery and technique. The regional anesthesia, injection anesthesia paradigm was now officially shifted, and the path made available for others to follow.[3]

HISTORY OF INTRAOCULAR ANESTHESIA

Mae West was once asked how she reached the pinnacle of her profession. Her reply, "I climbed the ladder of success wrong by wrong." Well, I might very well be wrong on this one, but to the best of my knowledge, the first published description of purposely placing an anesthetic agent into the eye was, again, by Fichman.[4] Again, to the best of my knowledge, Jim Gills, MD popularized intracameral Xylocaine at the 1995 American Academy of Ophthalmology meeting. Certainly many surgeons, including myself, began using it very soon thereafter.

Is Intraocular Anesthesia Really Necessary?

Just before he assumed office, Ronald Reagan was briefed by his advisors on the many problems that the country faced. He joked, "I think I'll demand a recount." Please know that there are many surgeons out there that feel the same way about intracameral Xylocaine. They just feel that it is not additive to the topical component and, therefore, it offers no real added value. They may use it under special circumstances, but for most surgeries, they go with topical only. I, on the other hand, am a strong proponent of intraocular Xylocaine and use it 100% of the time, even when I use the occasional block. For my money, topical and intraocular Xylocaine are truly synergistic. And, since I'm the one holding the pen, from this point forward I will present them as a team.

The Debate

Let's play pretend for a little while. Let's pretend that we are going to participate in a debate, the subject of which is "anesthesia for phacoemulsification: topical/intraocular vs. injection." This debate is unusual in that we are actually going to argue both sides. In preparation, let's make a list of all the advantages and disadvantages we can think of for both approaches. We'll start with the disadvantages—first injection, then topical—followed by the advantages.

Injection Disadvantages

Placing a needle somewhere within the orbit and then blindly injecting a liquid anesthetic carries with it many potential problems.[5-8] For the sake of drama, we'll start our list with those that are potentially life threatening or sight threatening (Table 6-1). Such frightening sequelae as cardiopulmonary arrest or globe perforation appear.

Keeping in mind that the best definition of minor surgery is "surgery done to someone else", there is also a category of "nuisance" side effects associated with this technique (ie, they may be "nuisance" to our patients, but we ophthalmologists have come to accept them as being part and parcel of injection anesthesia) (Table 6-2). Pain, fear, ptosis, diplopia… it's a pretty long list.

Topical/Intraocular Disadvantages

If you have never done it, the idea of doing phacoemulsification using only topical/intraocular anesthesia certainly conjures up a rather long list of potential disadvantages (Table 6-3). Squeezing, moving, pain, and anxiety for both patient and surgeon come to mind!

Injection Advantages

As in most facets of life, there is a real comfort for that in which we are familiar. Regional injection anesthesia is the well-established tradition in North American ophthalmology for cataract surgery. That comfort, that acceptance, is right at the top of the list for its advantages (Table 6-4).

Topical/Intraocular Advantages

It's easy to start the list of potential advantages of topical/intraocular anesthesia by simply noting that you can avoid all of the potential systemic and ocular disadvantages associated with injection anesthesia listed in Tables 6-1 and 6-2. However, we can go beyond those by realizing that, among other things, it is the quickest modality by which to return postsurgical vision (Table 6-5). That is particularly rewarding for the one-eyed patient.

Possibility vs. Probability

Now that we've got our lists, you've likely chosen the side you'd prefer to argue. For those of you who'd like to stay with injection anesthesia, I can almost hear you saying now, "Well, yes, it's possible that all those things could happen with a retrobulbar/peribulbar block, but, come on, the probability is quite low, especially the

Table 6-1

Partial List of Potential Life/Vision-Threatening Side Effects From Injection Anesthesia

Life-threatening

- CNS injection
  - Seizure
  - Pulmonary arrest
- Intravascular injection
  - Cardiac arrest
- Requires discontinuing anticoagulants

Vision-threatening

- Globe perforation
- Optic nerve perforation
- Retrobulbar hemorrhage

Table 6-2

List of Potential "Nuisance" Disadvantages from Injection Anesthesia

- Pain
- Fear/anxiety
- Prolonged visual recovery
- Temporary loss of depth perception
- Increased IOP
  - Need for oculocompression
- Ptosis
  - Temporary
  - Permanent
- Diplopia
  - Temporary
  - Permanent
- Subconjunctival hemorrhage
- Lid ecchymosis
- "Block head" feeling
- Need for patch
- Need for sedation
- Need for anesthesiology assistance
- Required to stop anticoagulants

Table 6-3

List of Potential Disadvantages of Topical/Intraocular Anesthesia

- Pain
- Fear, anxiety
- Eye movement
- Lid squeezing
- Corneal epithelial toxicity
  - Drops
  - Drying
  - Microscope light
- Loss of intraoperative flexibility
  - More difficult to deal with complications
- Painful if subconjunctival antibiotics/steroids injected
- Sensitivity to microscope light
- Physician must be willing to communicate with patient throughout procedure
- Patient must be able and willing to cooperate throughout procedure
- Physician must be facile with phacoemulsification
  - Must have short surgical times (< 20 mins)
- Cannot touch iris
- Must do corneal tunnel incisions
- Requires sedation
  - Need for anesthesiology assistance
- Immediate headache/brow ache if miochol, miostat injected intracamerally

really nasty ones. Besides, is a little bruising, etc really such a high price to pay for the safety of injection anesthesia?" Am I anywhere close?

Well, I can guarantee you that those of us who'd like to debate in favor of topical/intraocular anesthesia would have our own possibility vs. probability statement. When properly performed, there is always the possibility that items on the topical disadvantages list (see Table 6-3) could come true, but the probability of any of them happening is very low. On balance, our topical/intraocular team will gladly repeatedly evaluate and compare the advantage/disadvantage lists both ways. It gives us something to do as we prepare our anesthetic drops for the next case.

INDICATIONS, RELATIVE CONTRAINDICATIONS, CONTRAINDICATIONS

Simply put, the main indication for topical/intraocular anesthesia would be a routine phacoemulsification case. Now, to be honest with you, I have no idea what that means.

Table 6-4

List of Perceived Advantages of Injection Anesthesia

- Physician is familiar and comfortable with it
- Physician and patient can "disconnect" during the procedure
- Physician has more control over the eye
- Patient "feels nothing" during the procedure

Table 6-5

List of Advantages of Topical/Intraocular Anesthesia

- Avoid potential disadvantages of injection anesthesia
- Quickest return of postop vision
- For those capable, immediate return of normal depth perception
  - Less chance of stumbling, falling
- Retained ability to blink avoiding exposure keratitis/abrasions
- Less required time in pre-op area to become anxious
- Less cost
  - Decreased staff time
  - Fewer supplies
- Patient can "assist" during procedure
- Combines exceedingly well with the corneal tunnel incision approach

And certainly, a "routine case" may vary considerably from surgeon A to surgeon B to surgeon C. However, I need to commit to something, so here it goes. I am going to define a routine case as one in which the density of the cataract, the size of the pupil, the depth of the anterior chamber, etc, are such that the surgeon expects the case to go smoothly.

Relative contraindications would then be "nonroutine" cases. To me, that translates to circumstances that conceivably could take the surgeon outside his or her comfort zone. Once again, the comfort zone is going to vary considerably from one surgeon to another. Potential examples are as follows: extremely dense, black, "I can't believe I'm even trying this" kinds of cataracts, small pupils, weak zonules.

The contraindications are the easiest to identify. Anything that would prevent or disrupt good intraoperative communication and/or cooperation between the surgeon and the patient is, in my opinion, a contraindication to topical anesthesia.

Dr. Harry Grabow has nicely packaged these contraindications into what he calls the "Six Ds."[9] The first three are systemic in nature: deafness, dementia, and dysphasia (here meaning the inability of the patient to effectively verbally communicate because of either a neurological disorder or the speaking of another language). The second three are ocular and have in common the compromise of the patient's ability to reliably see the fixation light (the microscope light): dense cataract, degeneration of the macula, and dysfunctional ocular motility.

Attempting to identify the "personality profile" of the good and bad candidates is virtually impossible. Timidity, anxiety, and the "I don't want to feel or know anything," type of patient usually does quite well with topical anesthesia. The "I can take anything, Doc!" kind of patient might be less cooperative than originally perceived.

I will share with you, however, that I usually do not recommend topical/intraocular anesthesia for those individuals who are exquisitely sensitive (semicombative) to the light of the indirect ophthalmoscope during the preoperative exam. If the patient cannot tolerate that light, there is a reasonably good chance that he or she will not be very fond of the operating microscope light.

I do conduct the blood pressure cuff/lid speculum tests prior to commencing the case. Meaning, is if the patient makes a big stink about terrible pain and discomfort from either the inflated blood pressure cuff or inserted lid speculum, I will not even attempt to proceed with topical anesthesia. Anyone who is that sensitive to touch or pressure, in my opinion, would not perceive topical/intraocular anesthesia to be a pleasant experience. In well less than 1 % of the cases in which I encountered this sensitivity, I have simply decided to stop and administer a short-acting, low-volume, peribulbar block.

AGENTS/TOPICAL

Agents

The ideal agent for topical anesthesia would have the following characteristics: rapid onset, no toxicity, deep anesthesia, would always last as long as the case does, and could be instantly reversed if so desired. This ideal agent does not exist. However, there are some very good ones. I am aware of three commonly used agents: 0.5% Tetracaine, 4% Xylocaine, and 0.75% Marcaine. Proponents of each often say that theirs gives less corneal toxicity[9] and works better than the others. I've used them all and do not strongly endorse one over the other.

Because of my familiarity with 4% Xylocaine for topical anesthesia for refractive eye surgery, I have chosen to use it as my routine agent for cataract surgery (but, of course, the Tetracaine and Marcaine proponents will often cite the same rationale). I should point out, however, that liquid 4% Xylocaine is available in two different forms: the topical form and the systemic (injectable) form. The topical form is often used for mucous membrane surgery, as might be employed by oral and ear, nose, and throat surgeons. Ophthalmologists who use the injectable form as a topical agent for ocular anterior segment work often say that they feel more comfortable with its sterility. I use the topical form.

Xylocaine Jelly

More and more surgeons are switching from liquid topical agents to 2% Xylocaine jelly. It can be obtained as a sterile preparation from at least two sources: Astra makes a 2% Xylocaine jelly used by anesthesiologists for intubation, and Urojet makes a 2%

Xylocaine jelly for urological techniques. The Astra jelly comes in a 30 oz. tube that can easily be sterilely subdivided into smaller amounts, depending on how you wish to use it. It also comes in smaller 5 to 10 cc aliquots that potentially could be used as one per patient. The Urojet product comes in a 20 cc glass syringe that, again, can be sterilely subdivided. I prefer the Astra preparation in that I feel it provides the surgeon better vision.

There is a wide variety of ways that jelly can be employed. Some surgeons like to use it both in the holding area and as part of the preoperative preparation, some for the preoperative preparation only. I personally find it makes draping more challenging, so we apply a generous amount immediately after inserting the speculum. There's no doubt about it, Xylocaine jelly gives good topical anesthesia and serves as a wonderful lubricant for the cornea (the Astra preparation also contains hydroxypropylmethylcellulose), meaning that your scrub nurse will rarely, if ever, need to squirt the cornea. Besides, it's fun collecting those Flintstones glasses again.

AGENTS/INTRAOCULAR

The vast majority of surgeons doing topical/intraocular anesthesia use sterile, 1% non-preserved Xylocaine as their intraocular agent. Since the pH of commercially available Xylocaine is in the acidic range (6.4), some patients experience a burning or stinging sensation when it is first injected into the anterior chamber. For this reason, Joel Shugar, MD came up with a preparation that he cleverly calls "Shugarcaine."[10] He sterilely mixes one part 4% Xylocaine with three parts BSS Plus. This results in a 1% Xylocaine formulation at a more friendly pH and, perhaps, more endothelial cell friendly. Though, to my knowledge, no one has shown that the regular 1% Xylocaine is in any way toxic to living, human corneal endothelial. In fact, Gills[11] showed a 3% incidence of endothelial cell loss in his masked, randomized, prospective, parallel group study of phacoemulsification done with 1% sterile, nonpreserved Xylocaine—a number that compares quite nicely to phacoemulsification done without intraocular Xylocaine.

Systemic Medications

Naysayers of topical/intraocular anesthesia will often say something to the effect that those doing topical/intraocular anesthesia are "snowing the patients with systemic medications" and are really doing a form of semiconscious sedation. When topical/intraocular anesthesia is properly done, nothing could be further from the truth.

I have already stated that the main contraindication to topical/intraocular anesthesia is the inability of the patient to cooperate during the surgery. Therefore, significant sedation is not only unnecessary, it is counterproductive at best, and dangerous at worst!

For that reason, I have taken the liberty of adding "the seventh "D" to Dr. Grabow's six.[11] It is simply, "Drugs… just say no!" If the surgeon or patient can only attempt topical anesthesia by administering a lot of sedation, I would strongly recommend the surgeon continue the usage of regional anesthesia.

Now that is not to say that sedation of any kind can never be used. Topical anesthesia patients, like all cataract surgery patients, are about to undergo a new and different experience in unfamiliar surroundings involving their eye and their future vision. They are bound to be at least somewhat nervous and anxious. While much of that can be allevi-

ated by the demeanor, attitude, and communication techniques employed by the preoperative and intraoperative teams, I am not opposed to slowly titrated sedation for topical anesthesia.

We have found that, when needed, 0.5 to 1.0 mg of intravenous midazolam HCL
(Versed) works nicely the vast majority of the time. Many topical anesthesia surgeons are
fond of propofol (Diprivan), 10 mg (Diprivan comes as a white powdery substance, I've
heard it referred to as milk of amnesia).

In the unusual situation in which more sedation is truly indicated, do so in a slowly
titrated fashion. Remember, the goal in topical anesthesia is for everyone involved to be
relaxed, attentive, and cooperative.

TOPICAL/INTRAOCULAR ANESTHESIA, SCLERAL TUNNEL INCISIONS, AND CLEAR CORNEAL INCISIONS

One of the most prevalent misconceptions about topical anesthesia is that you have
to use corneal tunnel incisions. That is absolutely incorrect. When I first began topical
anesthesia, I was doing many more scleral tunnel incisions than clear corneal incisions.
Although the corneal approach is now, by far, my preferred technique, I still would not
hesitate to use topical anesthesia if I ever had to make a scleral incision again.

The simple truth is that you do not have to change any aspect of your current phacoemulsification technique in order to accommodate topical/intraocular anesthesia.
Bridle sutures, conjunctival peritomies, cautery, suturing, peripheral iridectomies, etc,
can all safely and comfortably be done with the topical anesthesia protocol I have outlined (see protocol section). In fact, that is the beauty of topical/intraocular anesthesia.
Physically, your routine does not have to change one iota. It is the mental change that is
the hurdle to topical anesthesia. Going to topical anesthesia requires a true paradigm
shift,[3] not only for the surgeon, but for the entire office and operating room staff.

While it is true that topical/intraocular anesthesia and clear corneal incisions marry
quite well, it is not a monogamous relationship. Topical anesthesia marries as well with
scleral tunnel incisions, combined phacotrabeculectomy, and trabeculectomy alone. In
short, it works well with small incision, anterior segment surgery.

I have no experience with planned extracapsular cataract extraction and
topical/intraocular anesthesia. Although I'm sure it could be done,[12] I personally would
be hesitant because of the tremendous amount of intraoperative control the surgeon
abdicates to ECCE.

PREOPERATIVE COUNSELING FOR TOPICAL/INTRAOCULAR ANESTHESIA

A question I often receive from visiting ophthalmologists seeing topical/intraocular
anesthesia for their first time is, "How do you inform the patient that he or she is going
to have surgery done with eyedrops only?" To that issue, I know of no better response
than that from Dr. Fichman himself, and I thank him for letting me share his thoughts on
this matter:

> "Patients in my practice are made aware of the fact that topical anesthesia will
> be used during their cataract surgery. The information is presented in a positive
> light, emphasizing the elimination of intravenous sedation and the general sense

that the patients will be up and at 'em almost immediately after surgery without pain, grogginess, or cosmetic deformity.

The patient is not encouraged to make a choice between topical anesthesia and regional blocks. The former is enthusiastically presented as the preferred method. Notably, many of the patients have sought out my services precisely to avoid retrobulbar or peribulbar blocks, or to regain vision immediately without the need of any eye patch.

One of my initial concerns in adopting topical anesthesia to cataract surgery was how to 'bring the patient along' as a partner in the venture. It was my feeling at the time, and one that continues after more than 1000 cases, that no purpose is served by telling an elderly patient that a controversial technique is about to be used requiring perfect fixation at the risk of substantial complications.

The fact that fixation during this procedure is almost natural is a difficult concept for the majority of cataract surgeons to fathom; in fact, the procedure's inexplicable ease is truly its beauty. If surgeons themselves are unable to fully appreciate the realities of cataract surgery under topical anesthesia, there is little reason to expect elderly patients, already apprehensive about the surgery, to assimilate the medical subtleties of the approach and feel comfortable in making an informed decision.

What appears on the surface to be ethical (an exhaustive informed consent emphasizing the novelty of the procedure and a reliance on voluntary eye movement, potential complications from noncompliance, etc) seems almost inhumane; ie, expecting an emotionally charged patient to make a rational decision on this point. Just as a prolonged informed consent regarding the benefits and risks of phacoemulsification versus planned extracapsular cataract extraction would be cumbersome and counterproductive, so also is a discussion of topical anesthesia versus local injection. The patient is not prepared to judge, nor should the patient be asked to judge, facets of surgery, such as phaco versus ECCE, two hand versus one hand, scleral flap versus corneal incision, one stitch versus no stitch, iris plane versus endocapsular, etc.

The onus for these decisions falls to the surgeon. Once the surgeon is confident that a particular technique is beneficial in his or her hands, the details become elements of the overall technique. It is a typical aspect of surgical medicine that a patient readily accepts all facets of the surgeon's regimen. Whatever the circumstances that brought the patient into the surgeon's care, the relationship in the preoperative period is one based almost entirely on trust.

Once I became convinced that cataract surgery with topical anesthesia was a superior technique, I naturally felt it imperative to communicate this belief to my patients. Our confidence in the overall quality of care we deliver—including the success and effectiveness of our anesthesia technique—permeates the patient's experience at my practice, extending even to the attitude and body language of the physician and staff."

Thank you, Dr. Fichman. I agree wholeheartedly.

PROTOCOL

Obviously, not every topical/intraocular anesthesia surgeon employs exactly the same protocol. My research, however, indicates that there are not major variants either. I am going to share with you our current protocol for topical/intraocular anesthesia,[13] and I will indicate, when appropriate, any interesting variation(s) of which I am aware.

PREOPERATIVE/HOLDING AREA

Tuberculin syringes (1 cc) are filled with fresh 4% topical Xylocaine. A syringe is assigned to each individual patient. The syringe itself serves as the dropper.

The patient's family and friends are encouraged to remain with the patient throughout the preoperative routine. A heparin lock is placed. If indicated, 0.5 to 1.0 mg IV of Versed is administered. The pupil dilating process is outlined earlier in this chapter.

No type of oculocompression device (eg, Honan balloon, super-pinky, etc.) is used. Topical/intraocular anesthesia has taught me that we create the need for these devices by placing a volume of fluid into a closed space.

Operating Room

The patient is transported into the operating room and placed onto the operating chair/table. Once comfortable and attached to the appropriate monitoring devices (blood pressure, pulse oximeter, cardiac), the preparation procedure is begun. First, the prep nurse, using the same 4% Xylocaine syringe used in the preoperative room, places several drops of anesthetic onto the appropriate eye. From that point forward, her prep is identical to that which we employ with injection anesthesia, with one significant exception. The prep nurse must now communicate with the patient, actually involve the patient, so that the feelings, sounds, and smells are not a threat but rather expected sensations. A drop of 5% povidone-iodine (Betadine) solution is placed into the inferior conjunctival fornix. This is followed by a routine Betadine skin prep of the lids, which is then removed with isopropyl alcohol and allowed to dry.

Immediately after the patient is draped and the speculum inserted, we place a generous amount of 2% Xylocaine jelly onto the eye. We try to cover all of the exposed eye.

The operating microscope light is turned down to its lowest intensity. I then make a big deal about announcing to the patient that the light is now coming and that, "at first it will seem very bright and I don't want you to be startled by it. In just a moment, you'll be very comfortable with it, but at first it will be quite bright." I then slowly bring the light onto the field and gently over the eye. With such preparation, rarely does the patient say anything. If he or she does, it is most often something like, "You're right, it is bright." By the time I'm ready for the capsulorrhexis, the patient is quite accustomed to the light; and thus, we turn it up to normal intensity for the remainder of the procedure.

We are now ready to proceed with the surgery. First, I make a sideport incision. I then inject the 1% Xylocaine directly into the anterior chamber through the sideport incision. For some individuals, this is accompanied by a stinging or burning sensation. Therefore, so as not to startle the patient and put him or her on guard before injecting the Xylocaine, I forewarn him or her with something like, "Mrs. Jones, I'm going to give you some numbing medicine now, and it might tingle a little." And, again, let me remind you of Dr. Shugar's "Shugarcaine," which takes the sting out of it altogether. How much should be injected? Everett Dirkson once offered these words: "I am a man of fixed and unbending principles, the first of which is to be flexible at all times." So it is with the Xylocaine. No set amount, just a few squirts will do the job nicely.

I then go through the following steps: exchange the aqueous with a viscoelastic agent, create the clear cornea phaco incision, do the capsulorrhexis, and then do hydrodissection with the same 1% sterile Xylocaine.

From this point forward, in general, I converse with the patient in order to: 1) remind him or her to look at the light, 2) acknowledge that he or she is doing a great job (he or she is a good partner), and 3) all is going really well. If I sense any level of discomfort, as might be indicated by a low groan, a little movement, etc, it is important to ask the patient directly, "Are you doing okay?" More often than not, what I learn is that either everything is just fine, that is just his or her normal breathing pattern/sounds, or that it is the inflated blood pressure cuff or pulse oximeter that is bothering him or her. If it is ocular discomfort, I employ verbal anesthesia to try to assure the patient that it is a normal sensation, that all is going well, and that it will soon pass. If indicated, we will slowly titrate intravenous sedation.

But, What If?

Okay, so maybe you can buy into topical/intraocular anesthesia for the routine, uncomplicated, smooth-going case. But, what if? What if something goes wrong? What if you get iris prolapse, need to enlarge the pupil, break the capsule, need to do a vitrectomy, drop the nucleus, drop the IOL, etc?

Fortunately, the answer is that you treat all of those circumstances in exactly the same fashion you would if injection anesthesia had been employed. In my opinion, it is not so much a matter of what you're doing, but how long it takes you to do it.

With the protocol I employ, I have found that I have about 30 minutes of good, comfortable working time. Once beyond that, my patients will usually share with me that they are feeling more than just pressure, it hurts! So, what to do then?

While theoretically it would be possible (and acceptable) to recreate a closed system using a viscoelastic material and taking advantage of the self-sealing incision (or sutures if necessary), one could always stop and administer a low-volume peribulbar block. Thus far, I have not found that to be necessary. I simply apply more topical drops or inject more Xylocaine. Be aware, however, that in certain situations (such as placing a secondary IOL in an aphakic eye, with an eye that had a previous vitrectomy, or with an eye with a broken posterior capsule) it is possible to have posterior diffusion of the intraocular Xylocaine that may lead to the anesthetizing of the neurosensory retina. This can give partial or profound loss of vision, which is the bad news. The good news is that it is transient.

Conclusion

I saw a great sign at a gas station the other day, "Kind and courteous self-service." Speaks volumes, doesn't it?

When something such as topical/intraocular anesthesia for phacoemulsification comes along, I believe it is our responsibility to study it, evaluate it, and judge as to whether it is serving, self-serving, or both. Can it represent a better routine approach to phacoemulsification for both the patient and the surgeon? Hopefully, my personal answer has come through loud and clear in this chapter. Like so many other advances in small incision cataract surgery, when properly understood, learned, and applied, topical/intraocular anesthesia offers many benefits to all parties involved.

REFERENCES

1. Williamson CH. *Cataract Keratotomy Course*. Baton Rouge, La. August 1, 1992.

2. Smith R. Cataract extraction without retrobulbar injection. *British Journal of Ophthalmology*. 1990;April:205-207.

3. Covey SR. *The Seven Habits of Highly Effective People*. New York: Simon and Schuster; 1989.

4. Fichman RA. Phacoemulsification and IOL insertion. In: Fine IH, Fichman RA, Grabow HB, eds. *Clear-Corneal Cataract Surgery and Topical/Intraocular Anesthesia*. Thorofare, NJ: SLACK Incorporated;1993:116.

5. Cionni RJ, Osher RH. Retrobulbar hemorrhage. *Ophthalmology*. 1991;98:1153-55.

6. Duker JS, Belmont JB, et al. Inadvertent globe perforation during retrobulbar and peribulbar anesthesia. *Ophthalmology*. 1993;April:519-526.

7. Edge KR, Nicoll JM. Retrobulbar hemorrhage after 12,500 retrobulbar blocks. *Anesthesia and Analgesia*. 1993;76:1019-22.

8. Zahl K, Meltzer MA. The complications of regional anesthesia. *Ophthalmology Clinics of North America*. 1990;March:111-123.

9. Grabow HB. Topical anesthesia for cataract surgery. Paper presented at The American College of Eye Surgeons (ACES) Annual Meeting. February 17, 1994; Ft. Lauderdale, Fla.

10. Shugar JK. "Shugarcaine" lessens burning sensation. *Ocular Surgery News*. 1998;1:13.

11. Gills JP. Intraocular anesthesia in clear corneal cataract surgery. In: Fine IH, Ed. *Clear-Corneal Lens Surgery*. Thorofare, NJ: SLACK Incorporated;1999:59-69.

12. Dillman DM. Topical anesthesia for cataract surgery. Paper presented at The Lennox Hospital Ophthalmology Meeting; March 18,1994;New York City.

13. Kuhn TS. *The Structure of Scientific Revolution*. Chicago, Ill: University of Chicago Press;1972.

14. Smith R. Cataract extraction without retrobulbar injection. *British Journal of Ophthalmology*. 1990;April:205-207.

15. Dillman DM. Topical anesthesia: How to get a good drop on your cataract surgery patients. Paper presented at The American Society of Cataract and Refractive Surgery Film Festival; May 9-12,1993.

7
Clear Corneal Incision Technique

William F. Maloney, MD

Clear corneal incision (CCI) is an increasingly important component of state of the art cataract surgery due to the inherent efficiency of this approach. Since its introduction, there have been three variations of clear corneal incision designs: hinge, groove, and single plane (Figure 7-1). All have been widely used by experienced surgeons with good results during the past decade.

When considering the characteristics of today's ideal CCI, it has been my experience that the single plane technique offers some potentially important advantages over those that incorporate a vertical groove. The groove often results in a foreign body sensation that can be more uncomfortable, last considerably longer, and in general, be more troublesome in the younger refractive patient who is typically professionally active. We now also know that it is the vertical groove component of the CCI that introduces the potential for surgically induced astigmatic changes. In effect, the groove (particularly the deeper 600 micron groove) functions as a peripheral astigmatic keratotomy incision to flatten the cornea in that meridian. In the typical cataract patient with against-the-rule astigmatism, this induced astigmatic change is often beneficial when the incision is located temporally. A temporally hinged incision is therefore sometimes used in cases with greater than 1.5 diopters (D) of against-the-rule astigmatism in combination with a peripheral astigmatic keratotomy incision placed nasally, with astigmatically beneficial results. It has been my experience that most other cataract patients (with 1 D or less of against-the-rule astigmatism) do best with the simple efficiency and astigmatic neutrality of the 3 mm single plane style of CCI.

THE SINGLE PLANE TECHNIQUE STEP-BY-STEP

The efficiency of the single plane approach derives from its simplicity. It is essentially a paracentesis that is 3 mm wide. The key to a fast and easy transition to this particular approach lies in proper blade orientation before the incision is made. Once those principles are clearly in mind, the incision itself is easy—simply think paracentesis!

Howard Fine described this approach and taught it to me several years ago. Since then I have used it exclusively in both cataract cases, and more recently, in clear lensectomy patients. The technique is as follows:

Figure 7-1. Of the three types of clear corneal incisions commonly used in cataract patients (hinge, groove, and single plane) I have found the single plane to be best suited to refractive lensectomy surgery because there seems to be less foreign body sensation and more reliable astigmatic neutrality when there is no vertical groove in the incision.

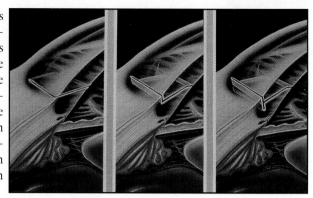

1. **Baseline blade orientation**
   Orient the blade so that it is parallel to the iris plane. This is the 0 degree (horizontal) plane. Then, imagine a vertical plane at 90 degrees for further reference (Figure 7-2).
2. **Blade position**
   Place the blade tip just at the start of clear corneal tissue. The anterior vascular arcade is a useful landmark. Now tilt the blade tip up and the blade heel down so that the blade is now on a plane of 10 degrees. This is the single plane that the incision will follow through the corneal tissue (Figure 7-3).
3. **Check for blade tilt**
   Confirm that the blade is oriented in such a way that it will remain perpendicular to the cornea as the incision progresses. Be particularly sure that it is not tangential to the cornea and that the blade is flat with both shoulders of the blade on the same plane (Figure 7-4).
4. **Single plane incision**
   The paracentesis is then created with a smooth, uninterrupted, straight-in, straight-out maneuver (Figure 7-5).

INSTRUMENTATION: DIAMOND OR METAL?

Typically, this incision has worked best with a diamond blade. The traditional metal blades are just not sharp enough to penetrate the external cornea cleanly enough to initiate this incision properly. This is another reason why many metal blade users began to incorporate a vertical groove to initiate the CCI. There is, however, a new generation of metal blades that are manufactured specifically for this clear corneal incision. They are much thinner and sharper than traditional metal blades and work very well for this single plane incision technique. Most blade manufacturers have a metal clear corneal blade now available or in development, and most offer some form of a free trial.

INCISION LOCATION: TEMPORAL OR ON AXIS?

In my experience, the incision is best placed temporally in the typical cataract patient. This location is most likely to be astigmatically beneficial to the typical cataract patient with against-the-rule astigmatism. Although attempts to neutralize preexisting astigma-

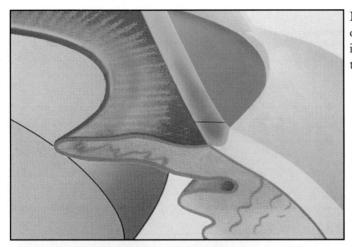

Figure 7-2. The baseline orientation for the blade is at the plane parallel to the iris, or 0 degrees.

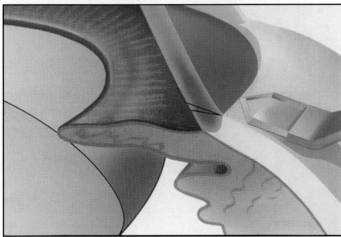

Figure 7-3. The blade is then tilted to align with the 10-degree plane. This is the single plane of the incision.

tism by locating the incision "on-axis" can sometimes neutralize small amounts of astigmatism in with-the-rule patients, astigmatism in these patients is usually more accurately corrected with astigmatic keratotomy. The improved access and visualization, which usually accompany the temporal approach, make the entire procedure safer and more efficient. This alone probably warrants use of the temporal approach in all cases.

INCISION SIZE

Although smaller is better when it comes to incision size, there is a point at which the incision is too small. An injected foldable IOL requires an incision of approximately 3.5 mm. Therefore, the typical 3.0 mm phaco incision needs to be widened with a blunt-tip keratome 3.5 mm wide, prior to IOL injection in order to prevent wound stretch and deformation. If the wound is not surgically enlarged, the resulting incision stretch can permanently deform the internal corneal valve upon which the crucial self-sealing capacity of this incision depends.

Figure 7-4. Check for blade tilt before making the incision.

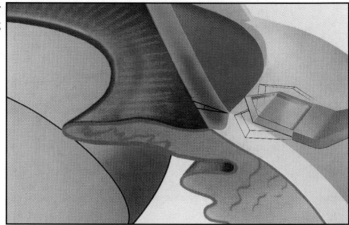

Figure 7-5. The incision is made as a paracentesis; straight in and straight out along the 10-degree single plane.

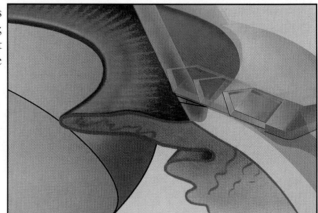

SUMMARY

Today's state of the art cataract surgery is a remarkably effective and efficient technique. Achieving the optimum results requires that we utilize the safest, most efficient, and most refractively accurate techniques at our disposal for each component of the procedure. Because of its inherent efficiency, secure self-sealing, lack of foreign body sensation, and its astigmatic neutrality, the single plane paracentesis approach is probably going to be the best choice for any surgeon transitioning to CCI at this time.

It has been my experience that refractive lensectomy patients do best with the security, efficiency, and astigmatic neutrality of the three mm single plane style of CCI. Any pre-existing astigmatism is addressed with separate, peripheral astigmatic keratotomy incisions either at the time of surgery or later at the slit lamp.

8
Anterior Capsulotomy and Cortical Cleaving Hydrodissection

R. Bruce Wallace III, MD
I. Howard Fine, MD

ANTERIOR CAPSULOTOMY

R. BRUCE WALLACE III, MD

Few innovations in modern cataract surgery have had a greater impact on surgical outcomes as has capsulorrhexis. We are indebted to Drs. Howard Gimbel and Thomas Neuhann, who independently described the capsulorrhexis technique over 10 years ago. Similar to sutureless incisions, capsulorrhexis gained worldwide popularity soon after its introduction.

A properly performed continuous curvilinear capsulorrhexis sets the stage for a successful cataract procedure. However, if a radial anterior capsular tear inadvertently occurs, the surgeon's confidence in the expected desired result diminishes. After a successful capsulorrhexis, Dr. Robert Osher commonly informs his patients that the "hard part" is over, and it is likely that everything will continue to go well.

The fallback procedures to unsuccessful capsulorrhexis include can opener anterior capsulotomy, avoidance of hydrodissection, two-handed iris plane phaco (described by Drs. Richard Kratz and James Little), and if the posterior capsule is compromised, insertion of the IOL into the ciliary sulcus. All of these maneuvers require the surgeon to work outside of his or her comfort zone, and the desired improvements in uncorrected vision can be jeopardized.

Considering the influence that a successful anterior capsulotomy has on achieving the best postoperative result, a dependable and reproducible capsulorrhexis technique is a major asset. Three adjustments to standard capsulorrhexis have helped me be more consistently successful.

"Soft Shell" Viscoelastic Technique

Described by Dr. Steve Arshinoff; two different types of viscoelastics are injected prior to performing anterior capsulorrhexis.[1] A thicker viscodispersive material, like Viscoat

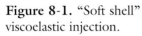

Figure 8-1. "Soft shell" viscoelastic injection.

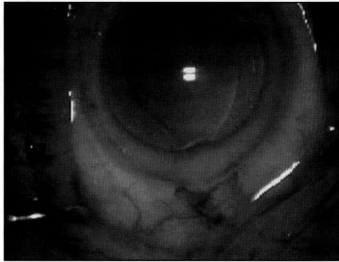

(Alcon, Fort Worth, Tex) or Vitrax (Allergan, Irvine, Calif), is injected first. Underneath this material, a second viscoelastic that is viscoadherent, like Amvisc, Healon (Bausch & Lomb, Claremont, Calif), or Biolon (Allergan, Irvine, Calif), is introduced (Figure 8-1). This additional viscoelastic material serves two purposes. First, it helps to drive the viscodispersive material toward the corneal endothelium for greater protection. Second, it creates a friendly anterior chamber environment to help the surgeon propagate and complete the capsulorrhexis without the resistance commonly encountered with a more tenacious viscodispersive material.

Improvements in Capsulotomy Instrumentation

Capsulorrhexis can be accomplished with a bent needle alone. However, there tends to be less surgeon control, particularly in difficult situations, such as with unexpected ocular movements or positive vitreous pressure. Completing the capsulorrhexis tear with newer capsular forceps that are contoured and thinner can provide more consistent results. A variety of forceps, almost all modifications of the original Utrata instrument, are now available, some with needle-like tips to initiate a central capsulorrhexis tear.

Globe Stabilization

With the advent of topical intracameral anesthesia, surgeons have faced the increased challenge of performing capsulorrhexis with potential ocular movements. Along with the use of capsulotomy forceps, the routine use of globe stabilization helps to minimize inadvertent radial tears with this less invasive anesthesia technique. Inserting a second instrument, such as a blunt cyclodialysis spatula, through a sideport incision reduces the risk of any sudden ocular movements, causing problems during the capsulotomy procedure (Figure 8-2).

Size of Capsulotomy

The best diameter for the anterior capsular opening is somewhat uncertain. Recent investigations suggest that a small overlap of the remaining anterior capsule onto the

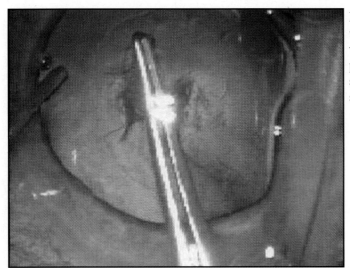

Figure 8-2. Completing the wider capsulorrhexis with globe stabilization provided by a cyclodialysis spatula through the side-port incision.

periphery of the inserted IOL optic may help to reduce posterior capsular opacification.[2] This means that creating an opening that is 0.5 mm smaller than the optic of the intraocular lens may offer the best long-term results.

Forceps capsulorrhexis allows the surgeon to adjust the size of the opening during the procedure. If the capsulotomy appears too large, simply changing the vector forces toward the center of the lens can redirect the tear inward. If the opening appears too small, the tear can be redirected outward, yet the surgeon faces the risk of a radial tear. One method to incrementally and gently expand the size of the capsulorrhexis is to use what I have termed "capsular lift." Once the surgeon realizes the need to increase the diameter of the capsulotomy, usually noticed about one-third of the way around the circular tear, the surgeon releases the capsular flap and with the forceps ends opposed, the tips are placed just underneath the advancing tear. The closed forceps are then used to lift the capsular flap, which moves the tear edge gradually outward (Figure 8-3). The advancing flap is then regrasped and the capsulorrhexis is completed with the new, larger diameter. For more information on anterior capsulotomy, refer to Chapters 10 and 11.

CORTICAL CLEAVING HYDRODISSECTION

I. HOWARD FINE, MD

Traditionally, hydrodissection had been the injection of balanced salt solution (BSS) into the cortical layer of the cataract. Fluid would circumferentially pass through the cortical layer and exit from the capsulorrhexis, leaving the firm cortical/capsular connections in the equator of the lens fully intact. In 1992, I published an article on a new method of hydrodissection, which I called cortical cleaving hydrodissection.[3]

In this technique, using a 26-gauge McIntyre cannula (Katena # K7-5150), the capsule is elevated in one of the distal quadrants and fluid is injected against the undersurface of the capsule in a gentle, continuous manner. The fluid goes circumferentially around the lens, between the cortex and the lens capsule, until it reaches the cortical/capsular connections at the equator of the capsular bag. This stops the fluid and

Figure 8-3. "Capsular lift" to widen the capsulorrhexis diameter.

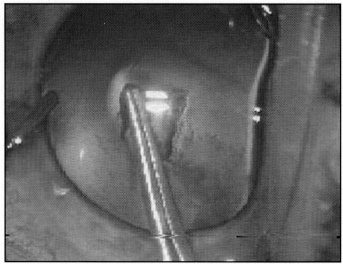

results in a trapping of fluid posterior to the lens complex. The trapped fluid elevates the lens, causing the capsulorrhexis to enlarge.

Once the fluid is trapped in that way, the same McIntyre cannula is used to depress the nuclear complex so that the posteriorly loculated fluid is forced to come circumferentially around the equator of the lens, rupturing the capsular/cortical connections and flowing out of the capsulorrhexis. This is accompanied by an immediate return in the diameter of the capsulorrhexis to the prehydrodissection size. Radial striations appear on the surface of the lens central to the capsulorrhexis as cortical fibers are washed centrally, with the fluid egressing from the lens capsule. The same maneuver is repeated a second time in the opposite distal quadrant.

During cortical cleaving hydrodissection, it is important not to depress the plunger of the syringe until the cannula tip has appropriately elevated the capsulorrhexis and anterior capsule. Otherwise, fluid will flow through the cortical layer, creating a path of least resistance, which will make it much more difficult to cleave the cortical/capsular connections.

Hydrodelineation is then performed, dividing the nucleus circumferentially into an endonucleus, an epinucleus with the cortex attached, and the capsule. Following removal of the endonucleus, the cortex is mobilized along with the epinucleus. This is performed by engaging the epinucleus distally in foot position 2, allowing the rim and roof of the epinucleus to occlude the tip, pulling the rim and roof centrally, and then going into foot position 3 and trimming the roof and rim of the distal quadrant of the epinucleus. With the clearance of occlusion as one enters foot position 3, the cortical fibers wash over the floor of the epinucleus and into the phaco tip. The floor of the epinucleus is reposited, the epinucleus is rotated 90 degrees, and the second quadrant is approached in the same way. Then, once again, the epinucleus is rotated and the third quadrant is trimmed. The final quadrant is rotated into the distal position. Using the roof as a handle, the epinuclear rim and roof are purchased in foot position 2 and pulled centrally toward the incision, while the second handpiece is used at the same time to push in the floor of the epinucleus away from the incision. This creates antiparallel forces, allowing the epinucleus to be flipped away from its proximity to the posterior capsule and to be mobilized with low powers of phaco or aspiration alone.

In the instances in which there is residual cortex (approximately 30% of the time), a dispersive viscoelastic (Viscoat) is used to viscodissect the cortex by injecting through the residual epinucleus against the posterior capsule in such a way that it elevates posterior cortical fibers and drapes them over the capsulorrhexis, while pushing peripheral cortical fibers further into the capsular fornix. The IOL is then implanted. The posterior cortical fibers, which are draped over the capsulorrhexis, fall back on top of the IOL and are easily accessible for removal along with residual viscoelastic because the cortical fibers are not attached to the capsular fornix.

In this way, I have been able to do away with irrigation and aspiration (I & A) of the cortex as a separate step in phaco surgery. I feel that this is an enormous advantage since a significant percentage of the capsules that are ruptured during phaco surgery are ruptured during cortical clean-up.

REFERENCES

1. Arshinoff SA. Dispersive-cohesive viscoelastic soft shell technique. *J Cataract Refract Surg.* 1999;25:167-173.

2. Hollick EJ, Spalton DJ, Meacock WR. The effect of capsulorrhexis size on posterior capsular opacification: one-year results of a randomized prospective trial. *Am J Ophthalmol.* 1999;128:271-279.

3. Fine IH. Cortical cleaving hydrodissection. *J Cataract Refract Surg.* 1992;18:508-512.

Phacoemulsification Technology: Improved Power and Fluidics

William J. Fishkind, MD

INTRODUCTION

All phaco machines consist of a computer to generate ultrasonic impulses, a transducer, and piezo electric crystals that turn these electronic signals into mechanical energy. The energy thus created is then harnessed within the eye to overcome the inertia of the lens and emulsify it. Once turned into emulsate, the fluidic systems remove the emulsate replacing it with balanced salt solution (BSS).

POWER GENERATION

Power is created by the interaction of frequency and stroke length. Frequency is defined as the speed of the needle movement and is determined by the manufacturer of the machine. Presently, most machines operate at a frequency of between 35,000 to 45,000 cycles per second (Hz) (Table 9-1). This frequency range is the most efficient for nuclear emulsification. Lower frequencies are less efficient and higher frequencies create excess heat.

Frequency is maintained by tuning circuitry that is designed into the machine computer. Tuning is vital because the phaco tip is required to operate in varied media. For example, the resistance of the aqueous is less than the resistance of the cortex, which in turn is less than the resistance of the nucleus. As the resistance to the phaco tip varies, to maintain maximum efficiency, small alterations in frequency are created by the tuning circuitry in the computer. The surgeon will subjectively appreciate good tuning circuitry by a sense of smoothness and power.

Stroke length is defined as the length of the needle movement. This length is generally 2 to 6 mils (thousandths of an inch). Most machines operate in the 2 to 4 mil range. Longer stroke lengths are prone to generate excess heat. The longer the stroke length, the greater the physical impact on the nucleus, and the greater the generation of cavitation forces. Stroke length is determined by foot pedal excursion in position 3 during linear control of phaco.

Table 9-1

Phaco Machines

Company	Model	Freq. KHz	Pump Type	Pump Comment	Vac. Range mmHg	Flow Range cc/min	Comments
Alcon	Legacy Series 20,000	40	Turbostatic Peristaltic	High vacuum pack	0-500	0-60	Flared ABS tip New software: burst/pulse mode
Allergan	Diplomax	40	Peristaltic	Microprocessor control of pump	0-500	0-44	Pulse/burst mode
Allergan	Prestige	47.5	Peristaltic	Microprocessor control of pump	0-500	0-40	Pulse/burst mode
Allergan	Sovereign	38	Peristaltic	Microprocessor control of pump Shield-fluid Coupled pressure sensor	0-500	0-40	Prosync on-board computer control. Power matrix and digital control Allows power down to 5%
Bausch & Lomb	Millenium	28	Venturi or Concentrix	Hybrid: programmable to emulate venturi or peristaltic	0-550	0-60	Dual linear foot Pedal modular upgrades
Mentor	SIStem	40	Peristaltic	Microprocessor control of pump Variable rise time (VRT)	0-500	0-50	Automatic surge suppression
Staar	The Wave	42	Peristaltic	Fluid coupled system	0-500	0-50	Surge suppression CD-ROM printout of events

ENERGY AT THE PHACO TIP

The actual tangible forces, which emulsify the nucleus, are a blend of the "jackhammer" effect and cavitation.[1] The jackhammer effect is merely the physical striking of the needle against the nucleus.

The cavitation effect is more convoluted. The phaco needle, moving through the liquid medium of the aqueous at ultrasonic speeds, creates intense zones of high and low pressure. Low pressure, created with the backward movement of the tip, literally pulls dissolved gases out of the solution, thus giving rise to micro bubbles. Forward tip movement then creates an equally intense zone of high pressure. This produces compression of the micro bubbles until they implode. At the moment of implosion, the bubbles create a temperature of 13000° F and a shock wave of 75,000 pounds per square inch (PSI). Of the micro bubbles created, 75% implode, amassing to create a powerful shock wave

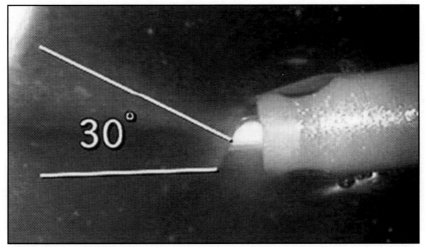

Figure 9-1. 30 degree tip. Enhanced cavitation shows ultrasonic wave focused 1 mm from the tip, spreading at an angle of 45 degrees.

radiating from the phaco tip in the direction of the bevel with annular spread. However, 25% of the bubbles are too large to implode. These micro bubbles are swept up in the shock wave and radiate with it.

The cavitation energy that is created can be directed in any desired direction; the angle of the bevel of the phaco needle governs the direction of the generation of the shock wave and micro bubbles.

A method of visualization of these forces, called enhanced cavitation, has been developed. Using this process with a 45 degree tip, the cavitation wave can be visualized and seen to be generated at 45 degree from the tip and comes to a focus 1 mm from it. Similarly, a 30 degree tip generates cavitation at a 30 degree angle from the bevel, and a 15 degree tip 15 degrees from the bevel (Figure 9-1). A 0 degree tip creates the cavitation wave directly in front of the tip and the focal point is 0.5 mm from the tip (Figure 9-2). The Kelman tip has a broad band of powerful cavitation that radiates from the area of the angle in the shaft. A weak area of cavitation is developed from the bevel but is inconsequential (Figure 9-3).

Taking into consideration analysis of enhanced cavitation, it can be concluded that emulsification is most efficient when both the jackhammer effect and cavitation energy are integrated. To accomplish this, a 0° tip, or the bevel of the needle, should be turned toward the nucleus or nuclear fragment. This simple maneuver will cause the broad bevel of the needle to strike the nucleus, which will enhance the physical force of the needle striking the nucleus. In addition, the cavitation force is then concentrated into the nucleus rather than away from it (Figures 9-4a and 9-4b). This causes the energy to emulsify the nucleus and be absorbed by it. When the bevel is turned away from the nucleus, the cavitational energy is directed up and away from the nucleus toward the iris and endothelium (Figure 9-5). Finally, in this configuration, the vacuum force (discussed below) can be maximally exploited as occlusion is encouraged.

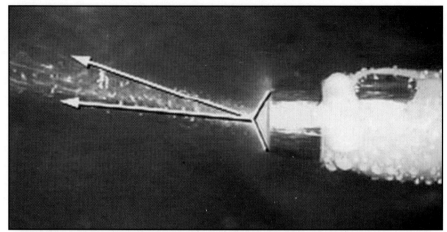

Figure 9-2. 0 degree tip. Enhanced cavitation shows ultrasonic wave focused 0.5 mm in front of the tip spreading directly in front of it.

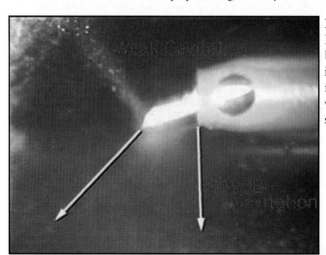

Figure 9-3. Kelman tip. Enhanced cavitation shows broad band of enhanced cavitation spreading inferiorly from the angle of the tip. A weak band of cavitation spreads from the tip.

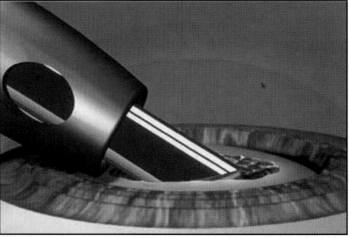

Figure 9-4a. 30 degree tip, bevel down.

Figure 9-4b. 0 degree tip.

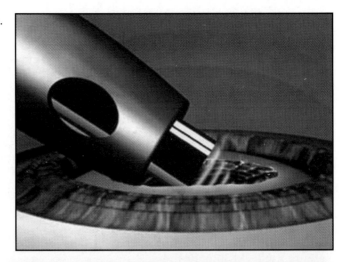

Figure 9-5. The bevel is turned away from the nucleus. Cavitation energy is wasted and may damage iris and endothelium.

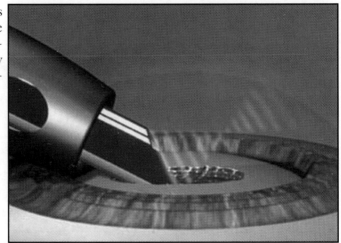

MODIFICATION OF PHACO POWER INTENSITY

Application of the minimal amount of phaco power intensity necessary for emulsification of the nucleus is desirable. Unnecessary power intensity is a cause of heat with subsequent wound burn, endothelial cell damage, and iris damage with alteration of the blood-aqueous barrier. Phaco power intensity can be modified by:

1. Alteration in stroke length
2. Alteration of duration
3. Alteration of emission

Alteration of Stroke Length

Stroke length is determined by foot pedal adjustment. When set for linear phaco, depression of the foot pedal will increase stroke length and, therefore, power. New foot pedals, such as those found in the Allergan Sovereign and the Alcon Legacy, permit surgeon adjustment of the throw length of the pedal in position 3. This can refine power

Figure 9-6a. Pulse mode in the Allergan Sovereign machine.

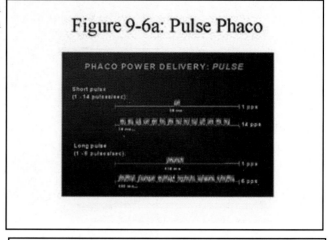

Figure 9-6b. Burst mode in the Allergan Sovereign machine.

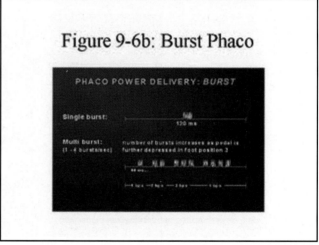

application. The Bausch & Lomb Millennium dual linear foot pedal permits the separation of the fluidic aspects of the foot pedal from the power elements.

Alteration of Duration

The duration of application of phaco power has a dramatic effect on overall power delivered. Usage of pulse or burst mode phaco will considerably decrease overall power delivery. New machines allow for a power pulse of a selected duration alternating with a period of aspiration only. In the Allergan Sovereign burst mode (the parameter is machine dependent) is characterized by 80 or 120 millisecond (msec) periods of power, combined with fixed short periods of aspiration only. Pulse mode utilizes fixed pulses of power of 50 or 150 msec with variable short periods of aspiration only (Figures 9-6a and 9-6b). Phaco techniques, such as the choo-choo chop and phaco chop, utilize minimal periods of power in pulse mode to reduce power delivery to the anterior chamber. In addition, the use of pulse mode to remove the epinucleus provides for an added margin of safety. When the epinucleus is emulsified, the posterior capsule is exposed to the

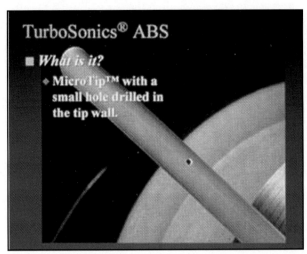

Figure 9-7. A 0.175 mm hole drilled in the shaft of the ABS tip provides an alternate path for fluid to flow into the needle when there is an occlusion at the phaco tip.

phaco tip and may move forward toward it due to surge. Activation of pulse phaco will create a deeper anterior chamber to work within. This occurs because each period of phaco energy is followed by an interval of no energy. In pulse mode during the interval of absence of energy, the epinucleus is drawn toward the phaco tip, producing occlusion and interrupting outflow. This allows inflow to deepen the anterior chamber immediately prior to the onset of another pulse of phaco energy. The surgeon will recognize the outcome as operating in a deeper, more stable anterior chamber.

Alteration of Emission

The emission of phaco energy is modified by tip selection. Phaco tips can be modified to accentuate 1) power, 2) flow, or 3) a combination of both.

Power intensity is modified by altering the bevel tip angle. Noted previously, the bevel of the phaco tip will focus power in the direction of the bevel. The Kelman tip will produce broad powerful cavitation directed away from the angle in the shaft. This tip is excellent for the hardest of nuclei. New flare and cobra tips direct cavitation into the opening of the bevel of the tip. Thus, random emission of phaco energy is minimized. Designer tips, such as the "flathead" designed by Dr. Barry Seibel and power wedges designed by Mr. Douglas Mastel, modify the direction and focus delivery of phaco energy intensity.

Power intensity and flow are modified by utilizing a 0 degree tip. This tip will focus power directly ahead of the tip and enhance occlusion due to the smaller surface area of its orifice.

Small diameter tips, such as 21-g tips, change fluid flow rates. Although they do not actually change power intensity, they appear to have this effect, as the nucleus must be emulsified into smaller pieces for removal through the smaller diameter tip.

The Alcon ABS (aspiration bypass system) tip modification is now available with a 0 degree tip, a Kelman tip, or a flare tip. The flare is a modification of power intensity and the ABS a modification of flow. In the ABS system, a 0.175 mm hole in the shaft permits a variable flow of fluid into the needle, even during occlusion (Figure 9-7). This flow adjustment serves to minimize surge.

Finally, flow can be modified by utilizing one of the microseal tips. These tips have a flexible outer sleeve to seal the phaco incision. They also have a rigid inner sleeve or a ribbed shaft configuration to protect cooling irrigant inflow. Thus, a tight seal allows low-flow phaco without the danger of wound burns.

Phaco power intensity is the energy that emulsifies the lens nucleus. The phaco tip must operate in a cool environment and with adequate space to isolate its actions from delicate intraocular structures. This portion of the action of the machine is dependent upon its fluidics.

FLUIDICS

The fluidics of all machines are fundamentally a balance of fluid inflow and outflow.

Inflow is determined by the bottle height above the eye of the patient. It is important to recognize that with recent acceptance of temporal surgical approaches, the eye of the patient may be physically higher than in the past. This requires that the irrigation bottle be adequately elevated. A shallow, unstable anterior chamber will otherwise result.

Outflow is determined by the sleeve-incision relationship as well as the aspiration rate and vacuum level commanded. The incision length selected should create a snug fit with the phaco tip selected. This will result in minimal uncontrolled wound outflow with resultant increased anterior chamber stability.

Aspiration rate, or flow, is defined as the flow of fluid through the tubing in cc/min. With a peristaltic pump, flow is determined by the speed of the pump. Flow determines how well particulate matter is attracted to the phaco tip.

Aspiration level, or vacuum, is a parameter measured in mmHg that is defined as the magnitude of negative pressure created in the tubing. Vacuum is the determinant of how well, once occluded on the phaco tip, particulate material will be held to the tip.

VACUUM SOURCES

There are three categories of vacuum sources, or pumps. These are flow pumps, vacuum pumps, and hybrid pumps.

Flow Pump

The primary example of the flow pump type is the peristaltic pump. These pumps allow for independent control of both aspiration rate and aspiration level.

Vacuum Pump

The primary example of the vacuum pump is the venturi pump. This pump type allows direct control of only vacuum level. Flow is dependent upon the vacuum level setting. Additional examples are the rotary vane and diaphragmatic pumps.

Hybrid Pump

The primary example of the hybrid pump is the Allergan Sovereign peristaltic pump (Figure 9-8) or the Bausch & Lomb Concentrix pump (Figure 9-9). These pumps are interesting in that they are able to act like either a vacuum or flow pump dependent upon

Figure 9-8. The Allergan peristaltic pump. Controlled by digital inputs it can move forward, backward, or oscillate, instantaneously.

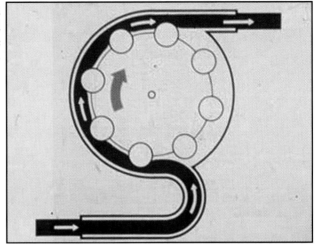

Figure 9-9. The Bausch & Lomb Concentrix pump. Inside two cam-shaped discs rotate to generate a vacuum that is regulated to emulate either a peristaltic or venturi pump.

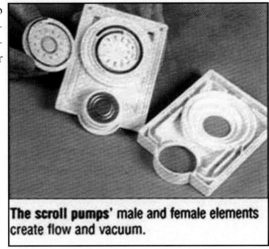

The scroll pumps' male and female elements create flow and vacuum.

programming. They are the most recent supplement to pump types and are generally controlled by digital inputs, creating incredible flexibility and responsiveness.

The challenge to the surgeon is to balance the effect of phaco intensity, which tends to push nuclear fragments off the phaco tip with the effect of flow, which attracts fragments toward the phaco tip and vacuum, holding the fragments on the phaco tip. Generally, low flow slows down intraocular events, while high flow speeds them up. Low or zero vacuum is helpful during sculpting of a hard or large nucleus, where the high power intensity of the tip may be applied near the iris or anterior capsule. Zero vacuum will avoid inadvertent aspiration of the iris or capsule, preventing significant morbidity.

SURGE

A principal limiting factor in the selection of high levels of vacuum and/or flow is the development of surge. When the phaco tip is occluded, flow is interrupted and vacuum builds to its preset level. Emulsification of the occluding fragment then clears the occlusion. Flow immediately begins at the preset level in the presence of the high vacuum level. In addition, if the aspiration line tubing is not reinforced to prevent collapse (tubing compliance), the tubing will have constricted during the occlusion. It then expands on occlusion break. The expansion is an additional source of vacuum production. These factors cause a rush of fluid from the anterior segment into the phaco tip. This fluid may not be replaced rapidly enough by infusion to prevent shallowing of the anterior chamber; therefore, there is subsequent rapid anterior movement of the posterior capsule. This abrupt forceful stretching of the bag around nuclear fragments may be a cause of capsular tears. In addition, the posterior capsule can be literally sucked into the phaco tip, tearing it. The magnitude of the surge is contingent on the presurge settings of flow and vacuum.

Surge is therefore modified by selecting lower levels of flow and vacuum. The phaco machine manufacturers help to decrease surge by providing noncompliant aspiration tubing. This tubing will not constrict in the presence of high levels of vacuum. More important are new technologies, which are noteworthy:

- Allergan Sovereign—Microprocessors sample vacuum and flow parameters 50 times a second, creating a "virtual" anterior chamber model. At the moment of surge, the machine computer senses the increase in flow and instantaneously slows or reverses the pump to stop surge production.
- B&L Millennium—The dual linear foot pedal can be programmed to separate both the flow and vacuum from power. In this way, flow or vacuum can be lowered before beginning the emulsification of an occluding fragment. The emulsification therefore occurs in the presence of a lower vacuum or flow so that surge is minimized.
- Alcon Legacy—The aspiration bypass system (ABS) tips have 0.175 mm holes drilled in the shaft of the needle. During occlusion, the hole provides for a continuous alternate fluid flow. This will cause dampening of the surge on occlusion break.

Phaco Technique and Machine Technology

The patient will have the best visual result when total phaco energy delivered to the anterior segment is minimized. Additionally, phaco energy should be focused into the nucleus. This will prevent damage to iris blood vessels and endothelium. Finally, proficient emulsification will lead to shorter overall surgical time. Therefore, a lesser amount of irrigation fluid will pass through the anterior segment.

The general principles of power management are to focus phaco energy into the nucleus, vary fluid parameters for efficient sculpting and fragment removal, and minimize surge.

Divide and Conquer Phaco

Sculpting

To focus cavitation energy into the nucleus, a 0, 15, or 30 degree tip turned bevel down should be utilized. Zero or low vacuum (dependent upon the manufacturer's recommendation) is mandatory for bevel down phaco in order to prevent occlusion. Occlusion, at best, will cause excessive movement of the nucleus during sculpting. At worst, occlusion occurring near the equator is the cause of tears in the equatorial bag early in the phaco procedure while occlusion at the bottom of a groove will cause phaco through the posterior capsule. Once the groove is judged to be adequately deep, the bevel of the tip should be rotated to the bevel up position to improve visibility and prevent the possibility of phaco through the posterior nucleus and capsule.

Quadrant and Fragment Removal

The tip selected, as noted above, is retained. Vacuum and flow are increased to reasonable limits subject to the machine being used. The limiting factor to these levels is the development of surge. The bevel of the tip is turned toward the quadrant or fragment, and low pulsed or burst power is applied at a level high enough to emulsify the fragment without driving it from the phaco tip. Chatter is defined as a fragment bouncing from the phaco tip due to aggressive application of phaco energy.

Epinucleus and Cortex Removal

For removal of the epinucleus and cortex, the vacuum is decreased while flow is maintained. This allows for grasping of the epinucleus to the anterior capsule. The low vacuum will help the tip hold the epinucleus on the phaco tip without breaking off chunks due to high vacuum, so that it scrolls around the equator and can be pulled to the level of the iris. Here, low-power pulsed phaco is employed for emulsification. If cortical cleaving hydrodissection has been performed, the cortex will be removed concurrently.

Stop and Chop Phaco

Groove creation is performed as noted above, under divide and conquer sculpting techniques.

Once the groove is adequate, the phaco tip and chopper are placed in the depth of the groove and separated, creating a crack. Vacuum and flow are increased to improve the holding ability of the phaco tip. The nucleus is rotated 90°, the tip is then burrowed into the mass of one heminucleus using pulsed linear phaco. The sleeve should be 1 mm from the base of the bevel of the phaco tip to allow adequate exposed needle length for sufficient holding power. Excessive phaco energy application is to be avoided, as this will cause nuclear material immediately adjacent to the tip to be emulsified. The space created in the vicinity of the tip is responsible for interfering with the seal around the tip as well as the capability of the vacuum to hold the nucleus. The nucleus will then pop off the phaco tip, making chopping more difficult. With a good seal, the heminucleus can be drawn toward the incision, and the chopper can be inserted at the endonucleus/epinucleus junction. The pie-shaped piece of nucleus thus created is removed with low-power pulsed phaco, as discussed in the Divide and Conquer section. Epinucleus and cortex removal is also performed as noted above.

Phaco Chop

The phaco chop requires no sculpting. Therefore, the procedure is initiated with high vacuum and flow and linear pulsed phaco power. For a 0 degree tip, when emulsifying a hard nucleus, a small trough may be required to create adequate room for the phaco tip to borrow deep into the nucleus. For a 15 or 30 degree tip, the tip should be rotated bevel down, to engage the nucleus. A few bursts, or pulses, of phaco energy will allow the tip to be buried within the nucleus. It then can be drawn toward the incision to allow the chopper access to the epi-endo nuclear junction. If the nucleus comes off the phaco tip, excessive power has produced a space around the tip, impeding vacuum holding power as noted above. The first chop is then produced. Minimal rotation of the nucleus will allow for creation of the second chop. The first pie-shaped segment of nucleus is mobilized with high vacuum and elevated to the iris plane. There it is emulsified with low linear power, high vacuum, and moderate flow.

Irrigation and Aspiration (I & A)

Similar to phaco, anterior chamber stability during I & A is due to a balance of inflow and outflow. Wound outflow can be minimized by employing a soft sleeve around the I & A tip. Combined with a small incision (2.8 to 3 mm) a deep and stable anterior chamber will result. Generally, a 0.3 mm I & A tip is used. With this orifice, a vacuum of 500 mmHg and flow of 20 cc/min is excellent to tease cortex from the fornices. The linear vacuum allows the cortex to be grasped under the anterior capsule and drawn into the center of the pupil at the iris plane. There, in the safety of a deep anterior chamber, the vacuum can be increased and the cortex aspirated.

Vitrectomy

Most phaco machines are equipped with a vitreous cutter, which is activated by compressed air or electric motor. As noted previously, preservation of a deep anterior chamber is dependent upon a balance of inflow and outflow. For vitrectomy, a 23-g cannula, or chamber maintainer inserted through a paracentesis provides inflow. Bottle height should be adequate to prevent chamber collapse. The vitrector should be inserted through another paracentesis. If equipped with a Charles sleeve, this should be removed and discarded. Utilizing a flow of 20 cc/min, vacuum of 250 mmHg, and a cutting rate of 250 to 350 cuts/min, the vitrector should be placed through the tear in the posterior capsule, orifice facing upward, pulling vitreous out of the anterior chamber. The vitreous should be removed to the level of the posterior capsule.

CONCLUSION

It has been said that the phaco procedure is a blend of technology and technique. Awareness of the principles that influence phaco machine settings is requisite for the performance of a proficient and safe operation. Additionally, often during the procedure, there is a demand for modification of the initial parameters. A thorough understanding of fundamental principles will enhance the capability of the surgeon for appropriate response to this requirement.

It is a fundamental principle that through relentless evaluation of the interaction of the machine and the phaco technique, the skilled surgeon will find innovative methods to enhance technique. "The road to success is always under construction."

REFERENCE

1.   Cimino WW, Bond LJ. Physics of ultrasonic surgery using tissue fragmentation Part II. *Ultrasound in Medicine and Biology*. 1996;22(1):101-117.

10 Phacoemulsification Techniques

William F. Maloney, MD
Louis D. Nichamin, MD
R. Bruce Wallace III, MD

SUPRACAPSULAR PHACO: A CAPSULE-FREE APPROACH

WILLIAM F. MALONEY, MD

Adding to the concepts comprising David Brown's "Phaco Flip" approach, I described a supracapsular approach to phaco in the *Journal of Cataract and Refractive Surgery* in 1997. I have been using the supracapsular approach regularly since January 1996. This chapter will review the relative advantages and indications for the various approaches to supracapsular phaco and describe the specific steps involved in each of these techniques.

Taking advantage of the larger 5 to 6 mm capsulorrhexis, all supracapsular techniques remove (at least partially) the nucleus from the confines of the capsular bag before phaco begins. The potential advantages of supracapsular phaco include the efficiencies associated with a significant reduction of capsular rupture and its related complications, as well as greater phaco efficiency due to the enhanced "nuclear followability," which can be achieved with the higher aspiration flow rates used with these capsule-free techniques. Significantly higher aspiration flow rates (typically one and one-half to two times higher than with endocapsular techniques) can safely be utilized outside of the capsular bag. Potential disadvantages have included the possibilities of mild postoperative corneal edema during the learning curve, as well as inadvertent iris contact with the phaco tip in cases with suboptimal pupillary dilatation.

Background of Phaco: 1967 to Present

Phaco has more or less reinvented itself each decade of its 30 years plus history. The most recent began right on schedule in 1996-97 with the supracapsular approach.

Anterior chamber phaco	1967-1977
Posterior chamber phaco	1977-1987
Endocapsular phaco	1987-1997
Supracapsular phaco	1997-2007

My 4-year experience with the supracapsular approach has taught me that when phaco (by any technique) is performed outside of the capsular bag, the entire procedure is more efficient. This efficiency results from three factors. First, greater access to the nucleus. Second, higher aspiration flow rates that can be safely used outside of the confines of the capsular bag. Finally, and most importantly, supracapsular phaco significantly reduces the most inefficient occurrence in phaco surgery today: capsular rupture and all of its associated potentially long-term complications.

Supracapsular Surgical Technique

In this section, three different supracapsular techniques will be described.

The preparation, anesthesia, and incision for supracapsular phaco are made according to the surgeon's preference (I recommend single-plane clear corneal incisions because of their efficiency), after which the following sequential steps are performed.

Capsulorrhexis

Viscoelastic of choice is instilled into the anterior chamber and supplemented as needed in a sufficient amount to maintain a flat anterior capsule throughout the creation of a 5 to 6 mm diameter continuous curvilinear capsulorrhexis (CCC) utilizing either cystotome or forceps. When creating this larger CCC, there is a higher chance of peripheral tears; therefore, a dispersive (more retentive) viscoelastic agent is helpful since it maintains a deep anterior chamber and thus a flat anterior capsule. Since peripheral tears are most often downhill tears that can occur when the anterior chamber shallows and the anterior capsule has become convex, maintaining a deep anterior chamber (AC) and a flat anterior capsule will reduce the chance of inadvertent peripheral tears.

Hydrodissection

A cannula of choice is used to perform cortical cleaving hydrodissection (as described by I. Howard Fine, MD) until the fluid wave is seen to pass beneath the full width of the nucleus and the lens begins to tilt upward through the CCC opening. If this spontaneous lens tilt does not occur, then nuclear rotation is utilized.

Nuclear Rotation

The hydrodissection cannula is used to gently rotate the nucleus first in one direction and then the other, assuring that the nucleus is free of all cortical attachments. Hydrodissection is then repeated. If, at this point, the lens again fails to tilt, the CCC is likely too small, and the supracapsular approach should be converted into any preferred endocapsular technique.

Lens Tilt

The lens tilt begins the process of moving the nucleus outside of the confines of the capsular bag. This is the point at which Richard Lindstrom's "tilt and tumble" phaco technique is begun (Figure 10-1a).

Tilt and Tumble Phaco

As described by Richard Lindstrom, the periphery of the tilted nucleus is emulsified in the iris plane using the classic two-handed phaco technique described by Richard Kratz. When the diameter has been sufficiently reduced (approximately 25%) the nucleus is flipped and further emulsified into a smaller and smaller single piece. The latter stage of

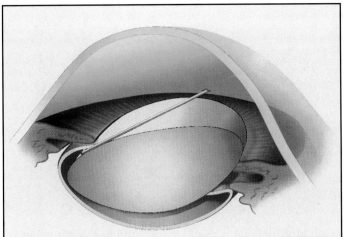

Figure 10-1a. Lindstrom's "tilt and tumble" phaco is begun.

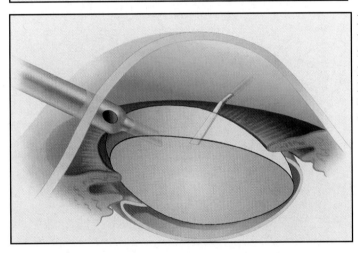

Figure 10-1b. The latter stage of the emulsification process takes place above the iris plane using higher aspiration for greater efficiency.

the emulsification process takes place above the iris plane using higher aspiration for greater efficiency (Figure 10-1b).

Nucleus Flip

The hydrodissection cannula is used to gently depress the posterior half of the tilted nucleus and then smoothly sweep the posterior equator across the posterior capsule until the superior equator is just beyond the vertical midline (Figures 10-2a and 10-2b). The hydrodissection cannula is removed (Figure 10-2c). This is where Dave Brown's phaco flip is performed.

Phaco Flip

The phaco tip remains almost motionless in the center of the anterior chamber and slightly above the iris plane. A Bechert-type spatula continually repositions the nucleus so that a fresh edge of the equator is repeatedly presented to the phaco tip. High aspiration results in very high followability as the nucleus is emulsified, almost nonstop, into a smaller and smaller single piece. Although the phaco process is twice as close to the

Figure 10-2a. The hydrodissection cannula is used to gently depress the posterior half of the tilted nucleus and then smoothly sweep the posterior equator across the posterior capsule until the superior equator is just beyond the vertical midline.

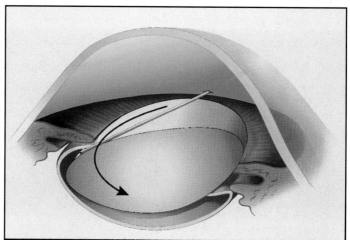

Figure 10-2b. The hydrodissection cannula is used to gently depress the posterior half of the tilted nucleus and then smoothly sweep the posterior equator across the posterior capsule until the superior equator is just beyond the vertical midline.

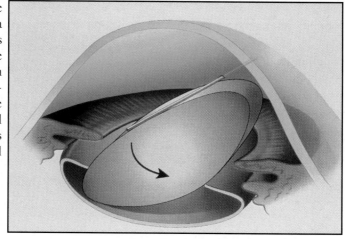

cornea, it is usually completed in less than half the time. Therefore, after the initial learning curve, the cornea is generally as clear with this technique as with the endocapsular approach, particularly if a more retentive viscoelastic agent is used (Figure 10-2d).

Inverted Nucleus Returned to the Posterior Chamber Above the Anterior Capsule

A viscoelastic cannula is used to continue to turn the nucleus until it is completely inverted and once again oriented horizontally. The inverted nucleus is then repositioned into the posterior chamber, below the iris, but above the collapsed capsular bag. Viscoelastic is supplemented as necessary (Figures 10-3 and 10-4).

Posterior Chamber Alternatives to the Supracapsular Approach

All of the usual endocapsular techniques (crack, chop, quick-chop, and prechop) can be used with the posterior chamber supracapsular approach. In my experience, everyone benefits from the increased efficiency that results from greater access to the nucleus as well as the enhanced followability seen with the higher aspiration outflow, which is

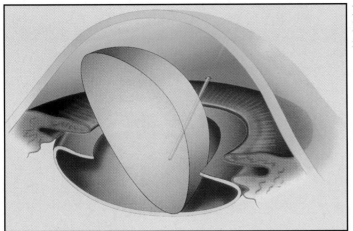

Figure 10-2c. The hydrodissection cannula is removed.

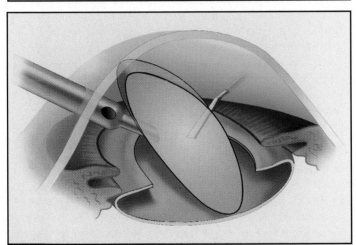

Figure 10-2d. The cornea is generally as clear with this technique as with the endocapsular approach, particularly if a more retentive viscoelastic agent is used.

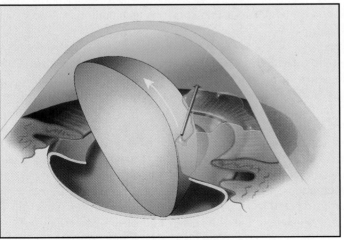

Figure 10-3. Viscoelastic is supplemented as necessary.

Figure 10-4. Visco-elastic is supplemented as necessary.

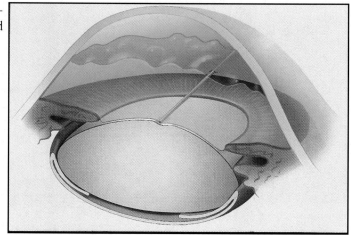

possible outside of the capsular bag. Flow-rate settings vary according to the phaco machine, surgeon preference, and the specific characteristics of the nucleus in each case. In general, my flow rates with supracapsular techniques have been up to two times greater than with the same techniques performed within the capsular bag. The most efficient posterior chamber method I have used is the quick chop technique taught to me by V. Pfeiffer, and also described by several other surgeons. I have found it most beneficial in cases with a very hard nucleus.

Phaco Quick-Chop

Cracking, chopping, and their combined variations require minor adjustments from their endocapsular versions. Without benefits of the anterior capsular rim to surround the disassembled nuclear components, I usually evacuate each disassembled piece immediately after it is separated. Followability is so enhanced, however, that I usually do not experience the very discrete sequential steps that I had been accustomed to with the more deliberate endocapsular approach. Otherwise the supracapsular quick chop phaco technique is really identical to the endocapsular quick chop technique that is now well known. The specific steps are:

1. **Phaco Tip Placement**

With a 30-degree phaco tip extended 1.5 to 2.0 mm beyond the irrigation sleeve and aimed directly toward the center of the nucleus, the tip is buried all the way up to the sleeve, which acts as a safeguard to deeper penetration. I have found the following machine settings to be helpful with tip placement: power adjusted to nuclear density with slow pulse mode of 2 to 4 pulses/second. This generally achieves a very tight fit between the tip and the nucleus. When the tip is properly placed deep into the central nucleus as illustrated, foot position two (aspiration) maintains the tight fit between nucleus and tip until the chop is complete (Figures 10-5a and 10-5b).

2. **Quick-chopper Placement**

The quick chopper (Storz #E-1103) should be in the AC before the phaco tip is buried. It is now placed immediately above the buried end of the phaco tip and the chopper tip is nestled into the anterior lens surface in order to gain a purchase. One end of this instrument is sharper for very dense nuclei, while the other is more rounded for moderate or soft lenses. You are now ready to perform the initial chop (Figure 10-6).

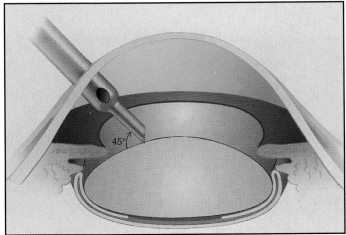

Figure 10-5a. When the tip is properly placed deep into the central nucleus as illustrated, foot position two (aspiration) maintains to the tight fit between nucleus and tip until the chop is complete.

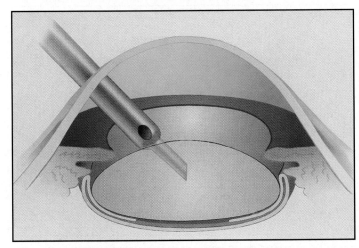

Figure 10-5b. When the tip is properly placed deep into the central nucleus as illustrated, foot position two (aspiration) maintains to the tight fit between nucleus and tip until the chop is complete.

3. The Initial Quick-Chop

The unique aspect of the quick-chop is that the nucleus is separated vertically, not longitudinally. This is accomplished by three maneuvers that, with experience, soon become one:

- The quick-chopper is depressed straight down (toward the optic nerve) (Figure 10-7a).
- The embedded phaco tip is slightly elevated. A central separation immediately appears (Figure 10-7b).
- The quick-chopper and phaco tip are separated laterally.

This last maneuver assures that the chop extends to full nuclear thickness and full length to both equators. Rotate the nucleus 90 degrees so that the chop is now horizontal. At this point, be sure of a complete initial chop by manipulating the two nuclear halves until a complete separation is confirmed (Figure 10-7c).

4. The Second Quick-Chop

The phaco tip is now directed into the middle of the wall of the inferior nuclear half, which is now exposed by the initial crack. The same machine settings as for the initial

Figure 10-6. The initial quick-chop.

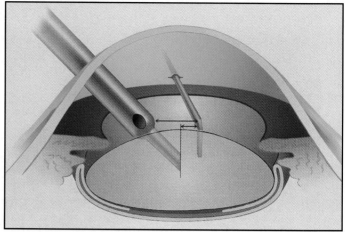

Figure 10-7a. The quick-chopper is depressed straight down (toward the optic nerve).

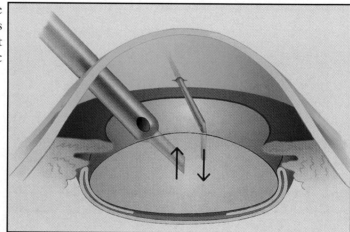

Figure 10-7b. The embedded phaco tip is slightly elevated. A central separation immediately appears.

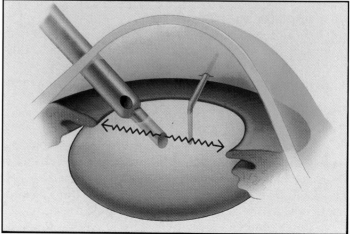

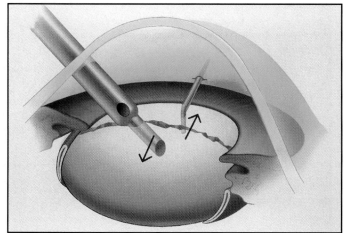

Figure 10-7c. Manipulation of the two nuclear halves until a complete separation is confirmed.

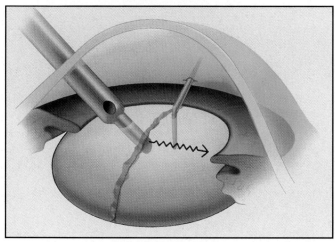

Figure 10-8a. Then, shorten the phaco tip extension to the more typical 1 mm beyond the sleeve and return to traditional linear phaco power control with aspiration flow levels approximately two times higher than is used for the same technique with the endocapular approach.

quick-chop are used. The chop of this inferior half is performed exactly as described above for the initial chop: quick-chopper down (80%), phaco tip up (20%), followed immediately by lateral separation until the separation is complete. Then, shorten the phaco tip extension to the more typical 1 mm beyond the sleeve and return to traditional linear phaco power control with aspiration flow levels approximately two times higher than I use for the same technique with the endocapsular approach (Figures 10-8a and 10-8b).

5. Sequential Nuclear Disassembly and Evacuation

The nuclear disassembly then progresses into smaller and smaller pieces as required by the nuclear density. Harder lenses are best divided into smaller pieces; soft lenses typically need not be divided beyond four quarters. In any case, I have found it best to evacuate each piece as soon as it is liberated when using the supracapsular approach, as the capsular bag is not present to keep the disassembled pieces gathered together while awaiting evacuation (Figures 10-9a through 10-9d).

Figure 10-8b. Then, shorten the phaco tip extension to the more typical 1 mm beyond the sleeve and return to traditional linear phaco power control with aspiration flow levels approximately two times higher than is used for the same technique with the endocapular approach.

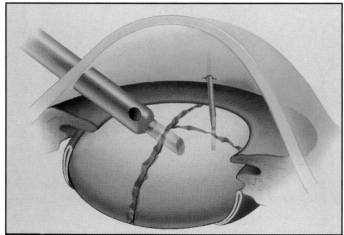

Figure 10-9a. It is best to evacuate each piece as soon as it is liberated when using the supracapsular approach.

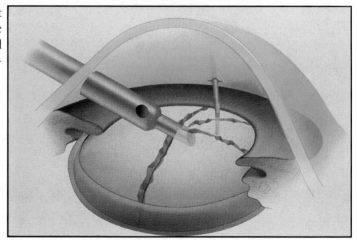

Discussion of Commonly Asked Questions

Patient Selection

Although I was very selective in my first year, I have gradually included all cases except for those in which the pupil cannot be enlarged sufficiently (either pharmacologically or mechanically) to perform the required 5 to 6 mm CCC. It is particularly noteworthy that once the maneuver of nuclear transposition is mastered, the supracapsular approach can routinely be used in pseudoexfoliation cases with excellent results.

Anesthesia Selection

I have used both injection and combined topical/intraocular modalities with equally good results. My preference is now for noninjection whenever possible.

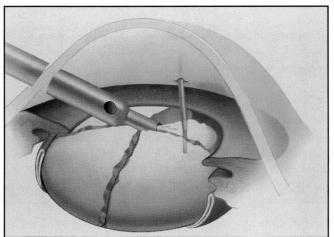

Figure 10-9b. It is best to evacuate each piece as soon as it is liberated when using the supracapsular approach.

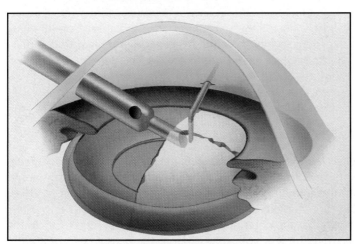

Figure 10-9c. It is best to evacuate each piece as soon as it is liberated when using the supracapsular approach.

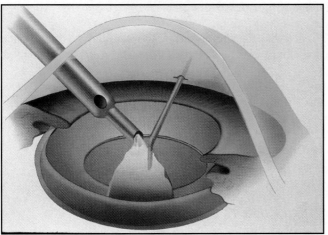

Figure 10-9d. It is best to evacuate each piece as soon as it is liberated when using the supracapsular approach.

Viscoelastic Selection

Although my experience has been primarily with Amvisc Plus, there has been no indication that the surgical maneuvers involved in supracapsular phaco would be in any way altered by selection of any alternative viscoelastic material.

Performing the Larger CCC

Although many surgeons already perform a 5 to 6 mm diameter CCC, most aim for a somewhat smaller 3 to 4 mm diameter, in part because it is easier to perform. Since I had become accustomed to the easier smaller capsulorrhexis, adjusting to the larger CCC was a significant part of my transition to the supracapsular approach. I found maintaining a deep AC and a flat anterior capsule to be the key. A smooth intact uninterrupted 5 to 6 mm CCC is a prerequisite for the supracapsular approach.

Hydrodissection

I have encountered subtle but important differences in hydrodissection when it is performed with the larger CCC. First, since there is a smaller anterior capsular rim to guide the fluid in the intended direction, slightly more fluid is generally required to complete the hydrodissection and subsequent lens tilt. Failure to achieve spontaneous lens tilt was almost invariably associated with a CCC less than 5 mm in diameter. In such cases, I routinely proceeded with an endocapsular approach. Most importantly, I learned never to attempt to transpose the nucleus unless the spontaneous lens tilt has occurred.

Is Nuclear Rotation After Hydrodissection of Benefit?

It is not unusual, especially early in the learning curve, to find that despite proper technique, the lens fails to spontaneously tilt. I encountered this situation regularly until I developed a better feel for the amount of fluid required for successful lens tilt. Needless to say, this is a crucial distinction, for excessive hydrodissection can rupture the capsule. However, studies have shown that the determining factor is the size of the CCC. In the presence of a 5 to 6 mm CCC, the lens will sublux before the capsule can rupture in response to prolonged hydrodissection. I developed the following approach when the lens does not tilt:

1. If the CCC is carefully inspected and confirmed to be the required 5 to 6 mm, and the lens is not inordinately soft, then the failure is likely the result of insufficient hydrodissection.
2. The hydrodissection cannula or a cystotome, if necessary, is used to gently rotate the nucleus clockwise 1 to 2 hours. The rotation is then reversed counterclockwise 1 to 2 hours until the nucleus is unquestionably free of any anterior cortical attachments.
3. The hydrodissection is repeated as above until the spontaneous lens tilt occurs.
4. If lens tilt still does not occur, an endocapsular technique of choice is performed. It is important not to persist with repeated attempts to transpose a reluctant nucleus.

Can Hydrodelineation Be Utilized?

I am familiar with the technique of hydrodelineation and have used it extensively with a variety of endocapsular techniques. Therefore, I initially attempted to incorporate this means of concentric division into the supracapsular technique in hopes that I could simply flip the endonucleus, and thereafter remove the remaining epinucleus. I was unsuccessful in flipping the endonucleus but, of course, it can very easily be subluxed into the anterior chamber and then repositioned.

Nuclear Flip

Provided that no attempt is made to force a reluctant nucleus out of the capsular bag, I am confident that this maneuver is the safest, most effective way to relocate the nucleus out of the capsular bag. There is ample clearance of the corneal endothelium that is further protected by the viscoelastic material. If the nuclear flip does not occur effortlessly, one can attempt to sublux the nucleus or simply turn to the endocapsular alternative.

Corneal Clarity Postoperative

Initially, during my first 3 months and approximately 100 cases, my corneas were not as clear as with my endocapsular approach. I experienced mild to moderate corneal edema that was proportional to nuclear density. Most cases cleared with extra topical steroid within 3 days. All cleared within 1 week. I suspect this is part of the normal learning curve for any supracapsular technique.

Why Should I Consider Supracapsular? What is the Benefit?

The benefits of increased efficiency, a wider variety of phaco options, and less phaco time can be expected to result from a transition to supracapsular phaco. However, the greatest benefit is the reduction in the incidence of capsular rupture. My experience has taught me that the most efficient location for the phaco process in the current post-viscoelastic era is outside of the capsular bag.

PHACO QUICK-CHOP

Louis D. Nichamin, MD

Since the introduction of traditional phaco chop by Dr. Kunihiro Nagahara, many variations have been described. In my experience, the safest and most efficient refinement is the phaco quick-chop technique, a term coined by Dr. David Dillman. Actually, this variation was described contemporaneously by several authors, including Dr. Thomas Neuhann of Germany, Dr. Abhay Vasavada of India, and Dr. Vladimir Pfiefer of Slovenia. Dr. Fukasaku's snap and split variation is also quite similar. The modification that these techniques share involves the location and placement of the manual chop instrument. Rather than making an excursion out to and around the equator of the lens, the manipulator is pressed down onto the anterior surface of the nucleus at a point just in front of or to the side of the impaled phaco tip.

This technique is becoming increasingly popular among surgeons who first attempted the traditional phaco chop, but found it to be awkward and potentially dangerous, since placement of the chop instrument out to the periphery and under the anterior capsule can be a somewhat difficult maneuver to visualize. The subtle refinement of quick-chop permits efficient division of soft, medium, and very hard lenses. Furthermore, it works well with small pupil cases and in eyes in which a generous capsulorrhexis cannot be obtained.

Figure 10-10. Vertical quick-chop initiated following deep impaling of the nucleus with the phaco needle.

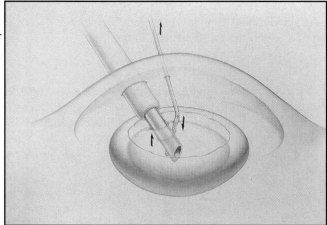

Figure 10-11. After the vertical motion, the instruments are separated laterally, propagating the division plane.

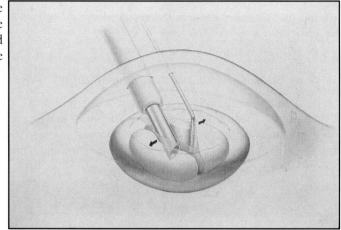

The procedure begins exactly as any phaco chop technique would. The central nucleus is deeply impaled using short bursts of pulsed phaco energy, along with a steep angle of attack into the central lens substance. It helps to retract the silicone sleeve, exposing more of the metal needle in order to maximize a deep purchase. The chop instrument is then placed just in front of, or to the side of, the buried phaco needle. Using the sideport incision as a fulcrum, the distal tip of the chop instrument is then pressed downward, assertively, into the nucleus as the phaco tip provides countertraction and a small degree of upward movement (Figure 10-10). As the cleavage plane is created, the chop instrument and phaco tip are spread laterally apart, propagating the division entirely across the nucleus from one pole to the other, as well as down and through the posterior nuclear plate (Figure 10-11). It is extremely important to verify that each successive cleavage plane is completely through the lens. One should not progress to the next chop unless this has been carefully verified.

The lens is then rotated, reimpaled, and the vertical down chop repeated (Figure 10-12). The more dense the lens, the greater the number of cleavage planes that are created. Once a section is chopped, the manipulator is used to push the chopped segment out toward the fornix of the capsular bag, causing the posterior apical portion of the

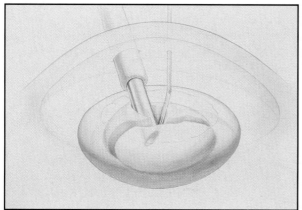

Figure 10-12. This process is repeated to create "bite-sized" nuclear segments for phacoaspiration.

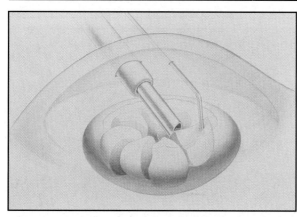

Figure 10-13a. Purchase of chopped segments is facilitated by pushing peripherally with the chop instrument.

chopped segment to present upward for easier purchase with the phaco tip (Figures 10-13a and 10-13b). High levels of vacuum and flow rate are used to evacuate these segments, and are aided by short bursts of pulsed phaco energy in order to collapse the nuclear material into the phaco tip. Purchase of chopped segments may also be facilitated by rotating the phaco instrument around its long axis to allow parallel alignment of the needle's bevel with the surface or facet of the nuclear segment, thus improving occlusion (Figures 10-14a and 10-14b). As the purchased nuclear segment is drawn centrally from the capsular fornix, it may be further subdivided utilizing traditional (horizontal) maneuvers, creating small "bite-sized" fragments which are more easily aspirated.

Several additional points should be stressed. As with any endocapsular technique, excellent hydrodissection is mandatory. An optional hydrostep—hydrodelineation—may be employed to create a concentric division plane between the hard inner endonucleus and the soft outer epinucleus. Working within the cushioned confines of the epinucleus may serve to increase the safety of the procedure. Also, chopping of an endonucleus allows for creation of smaller segments of nucleus, which make subsequent purchase and removal easier. Evacuation of the epinucleus, as taught by Dr. Howard Fine, is performed by gradually debulking and trimming the epinuclear rim until it spontaneously collapses in upon itself and is aspirated with little, if any, phaco energy.

Choice of the chop instrument is also important. With the traditional Nagahara phaco chop, many surgeons prefer using a chopper that incorporates a blunt or bulbous distal

Figure 10-13b. Sliding of the posterior apical portion up to the phaco tip.

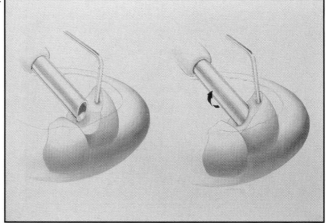

Figure 10-14a. Rotation of phaco needle bevel to appose chopped segments.

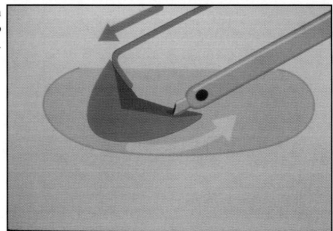

Figure 10-14b. Parallel alignment of bevel to nuclear segments improves occlusion and purchase.

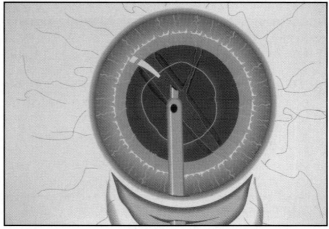

tip to increase safety when passing the instrument out to the periphery. With the phaco quick-chop technique, a more pointed, beveled, or flattened tip will more easily impregnate itself into the lens material.

When faced with a rock-hard nucleus, central sculpting or debulking is helpful. This will allow the initial quick chop to be carried out on a less substantive mass of lens material. Therefore it requires less mechanical energy and, hence, imparts less trauma to what is often a tenuous capsule and zonular network.

In summary, the phaco quick-chop technique is quickly becoming the preferred approach for nuclear disassembly by many surgeons because of its inherent safety and remarkable efficiency. It is applicable to most lens densities encountered and enjoys a relatively quick and facile learning curve.

BURST HEMIFLIP

R. BRUCE WALLACE III, MD

Burst hemiflip is a phaco technique that combines the beneficial elements of divide and conquer with the efficiency of nuclear flipping.[1] The idea of hemiflip phacoemulsification is not new. However, prior to the availability of recent generation phaco machines, many surgeons found flipping the heminucleus through an intact capsulorrhexis a difficult and unpredictable maneuver. This is probably why divide and conquer evolved into quartering the nucleus prior to nuclear removal.

Improvements in phacofluidics, especially burst phaco, has now allowed us to safely and more consistently flip or tumble nuclear halves into the iris plane prior to evacuation.

Hydrodissection

Like most phaco procedures, burst hemiflip starts with careful and complete hydrodissection of the nucleus. I consider Howard Fine's cortical cleaving hydrodissection to be the best method of releasing the nucleus and cortex from its capsular attachments. Properly performed, this technique allows for free movement of nucleus and cortex within the capsular bag. An added benefit is that cortical cleaving sets the stage for near total removal of the cortex after phacoemulsification. The surgeon can then proceed directly to IOL insertion, removing any small strands of remaining cortex while using the I & A instrument to evacuate the viscoelastic agent introduced prior to IOL implantation.

I languished for years trying to consistently perform this technique until Dr. William Maloney explained how I could improve my technique. He suggested that no pressure be placed on the syringe plunger when introducing the hydrodissection cannula into the anterior chamber. By keeping the thumb off the plunger, the surgeon is less likely to begin a fluid wave between the nucleus and cortex. Once the surgeon is certain that the tip of the hydrodissection cannula is just under the anterior capsular flap, a stream of BSS is carefully injected around the peripheral cortex, sometimes requiring multiple injection sites. Free spinning of the nucleus and cortex should now be possible. If there is resistance, hydrodissection should be repeated.

Figure 10-15. Separating the nucleus into halves.

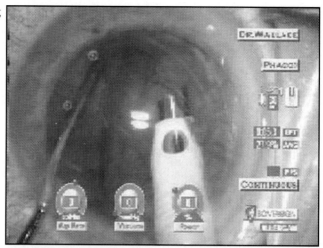

Figure 10-16. The first hemi-nucleus is flipped into the iris plane with bursts of phaco energy.

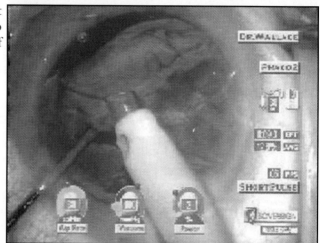

Nuclear Removal

To begin phacoemulsification, the irrigating phaco tip is inserted through the self-sealing phaco incision, and deep sculpting in phaco mode I is used to create a linear groove through the central nucleus. Similar to the standard divide and conquer technique, the two nuclear halves are separated with the use of two instruments, such as the phaco tip and a blunt cyclodialysis spatula (introduced through a separate sideport incision) (Figure 10-15). It is important that there be complete separation of the heminucleus. I have found that any residual attachments of the nuclear halves make hemiflipping difficult. The fluidics are now changed to phaco mode II and burst mode. With the separated nucleus still in the posterior chamber, the opened beveled port of the phaco tip now engages the top one-third of one of the nuclear halves. The phaco foot pedal is gradually depressed to initiate bursts of phaco energy, to generate a controlled flip of the nuclear hemisection, and to flip the entire nuclear half into the iris plane (Figure 10-16). This half is then emulsified while a second instrument is used to feed nuclear material to the centrally placed phaco tip (Figure 10-17). The other nuclear half is then spun into position and flipped in a similar manner and emulsified (Figure 10-18).

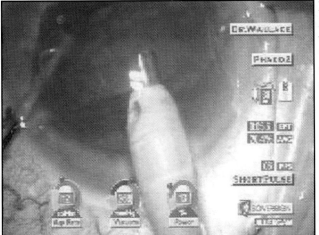

Figure 10-17. The first hemi-nucleus is emulsified while a second instrument "feeds" nuclear material to the centrally placed phaco tip.

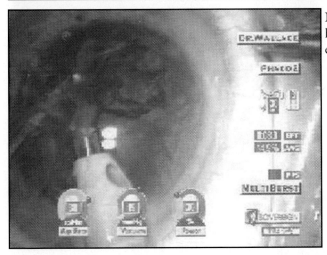

Figure 10-18. The second hemi-nucleus is flipped and emulsified.

Burst hemiflip works best for soft to medium hard nuclei. Very dense nuclei are probably best removed with quadrant divide and conquer or phaco chop.

Burst hemiflip is less challenging than full nuclear flips and not as likely to disturb the capsule, zonules, or corneal endothelium. By working further from the posterior capsule, there is less chance for capsular rupture and vitreous loss. I have found burst hemiflip phacoemulsification to be more efficient than quadrant divide and conquer and phaco chop for most cataracts.

REFERENCE

1.   Wallace RB. New phaco method marries opposing surgical methods. *Ocular Surgery News*. 1999;10:12-13.

11

Phacoemulsification in High Risk Cases

David F. Chang, MD

A well-centered posterior chamber IOL is a prerequisite for multifocal pseudophakia. Good centration is best assured by in-the-bag placement of both haptics, and a capsulorrhexis sized slightly smaller than the optic diameter so that its edge is on the optic surface. This avoids the potential decentering force of asymmetric capsule fibrosis that develops wherever the anterior and posterior capsule come into contact. If the lens must be placed in the sulcus because of posterior capsule rupture, capsulorrhexis capture of the optic may provide the best centration. Thus, if a multifocal IOL is planned, there is an extra premium placed upon preservation of an intact capsulorrhexis and an intact posterior capsule.

Failure to achieve these goals is more likely in complicated cases. For the purpose of this chapter, "high risk" refers to eyes with anatomic features that increase the chance of either a torn capsulorrhexis or posterior capsule. To avoid complications in these eyes, it is important to understand the mechanisms by which capsule problems occur. Factors which predispose an eye to capsulorrhexis complications or posterior capsule complications will be discussed separately.

CAPSULORRHEXIS RISK FACTORS

In addition to trapping the IOL haptics in the bag, the capsulorrhexis renders the capsular bag more resistant to tearing.[1] With forces such as cracking, a capsulorrhexis stretches like an elastic waistband without tearing. A single radial tear is precarious, however, because all of the stress placed upon the capsule is transmitted to that single weak point. Enough force will cause an anterior radial tear to extend around the equator into the posterior capsule.

There are four general conditions that increase the risk of developing a radial tear in the capsulorrhexis: poor visibility, eye movement, chamber shallowing, and increased capsular elasticity. These conditions may arise either because of the ocular anatomy or because of poor surgical technique.

Poor Visibility

A good red reflex is necessary for optimal visualization of the capsule. This is important in order to guide the flap and to monitor the direction of the tear as it develops. Delayed recognition of a peripherally escaping tear may preclude any chance to redirect it in time.

Ocular causes of a poor red reflex include tear film debris, decreased corneal clarity, small pupils, anterior cortical opacity (spokes), nuclear opacity (brunescence), and vitreous opacities such as asteroid hyalosis or hemorrhage. At the extreme, the red reflex is absent in mature white cataracts. Errors in surgical technique may also compromise visibility. Excessive drying or anesthetic can cloud the corneal epithelium. Poor run off of irrigation fluid may submerge the cornea. The capsulotomy needle can stir up the anterior epinucleus by penetrating too deeply. Finally, faulty instrument maneuvers may create cornea striae or displace the globe out of optimal microscope alignment.

Eye Movement

Lack of akinesia is characteristic of topical anesthesia or may be the unintentional consequence of a poor regional block. In this situation, performing the capsulorrhexis requires good fixation and cooperation on the patient's part. Sudden, unanticipated head or eye movement may result in a peripheral radial tear.

Patients must be properly selected for topical anesthesia, and cooperation is enhanced by appropriate levels of sedation and communication. Fixation is improved by avoiding excessive microscope light intensity, which can induce squeezing. During the capsulotomy, the cornea should be moistened in a way that prevents startling of the patient or surgeon.

Anterior Chamber (AC) Shallowing

The natural anterior convexity of the lens tends to steer any tear toward the periphery. The shallower the chamber, the more convex the anterior capsule becomes, and the more the tear tends to run centrifugally "downhill." The direction of the tear is best controlled if the anterior capsule surface is flat.

The most common cause of anterior capsule convexity is intraoperative AC shallowing due to egress of fluid or viscoelastic through the wound. Excessive instrument pressure on the posterior incision lip will burp out fluid through a momentary wound gape. Interrupting the capsulotomy to refill the anterior chamber with viscoelastic is important in this situation. A shallow AC may also be the natural result of a small globe or intumescent lens.

Capsular Elasticity

The more elastic a material, the more difficult it is to control how it tears. As an example, latex is more difficult to tear than paper. When an elastic material tears, it first stretches before abruptly splitting. Because of the rebound energy, the resulting tear is overly rapid and tends to advance away from, rather than toward, the grasping instrument. Because pediatric anterior capsules are very elastic, these capsulorrhexes are among the most difficult to achieve. The adult posterior capsule has less tensile strength and is more elastic than the anterior capsule. Accomplishing a posterior capsulorrhexis is more challenging because of this.

Two conditions give rise to what could be called "pseudoelasticity" of the anterior capsule. The first is poor surgical technique, whereby the capsular flap is allowed to become too long. The farther the capsule forceps are from the tearing point, the more pliant the flap becomes and the more difficult it is to direct the tear. If this starts to happen, the flap must be regrasped closer to the leading edge of the tear.

Pseudoelasticity also results from zonular laxity. Lacking sufficient circumferential tension, a capsule that is not taut will exhibit elastic properties. Such zonular weakness may first become apparent during initiation of the capsulorrhexis. If the anterior capsule is very lax, the capsulotomy needle tip will tend to dimple it rather than immediately puncture it. Next, as the capsular flap is pulled, the entire lens capsule may decenter from lack of zonular fixation. As with an elastic material, the capsular flap seems to stretch before suddenly tearing toward the periphery. Weak zonules are more common in eyes with exfoliation, advanced age, a history of retinopathy or prematurity, Marfan syndrome, blunt trauma, or prior surgery (eg, vitrectomy or trabeculotomy).

STRATEGIES FOR THE DIFFICULT CAPSULORRHEXIS

Visualization and control of the tear must be optimized in the high risk case. These same objectives apply to redirecting and rescuing a peripherally escaping tear. Although many of these principles are part of the basic capsulorrhexis technique, they are far more critical when dealing with a difficult case.

1. Maintain a deep anterior chamber. Frequent replacement of viscoelastic may be necessary depending on how much escapes through the wound. While attempting to rescue a peripherally escaping tear, pushing the nucleus posteriorly with a second instrument, as described by Dr. Christopher Conner, using the Conner Wand (Rhein Medical, Tampa Fla), can make the anterior capsule more concave. Cohesive viscoelastics perform better than dispersive viscoelastics in flattening the anterior capsule surface. A maximally cohesive viscoelastic, such as Healon GV or Healon V, may be necessary with narrow angles and a shallow anterior chamber. Rarely, an eye may have a nearly flat anterior chamber that cannot be deepened with viscoelastic. This not only makes the capsulorrhexis difficult, but may not allow enough room to mechanically stretch or enlarge the pupil. This also increases the proximity of the phaco tip to the endothelium during nuclear emulsification. In such cases, a mechanical pars plana vitreous tap may be necessary to achieve a sufficiently deep anterior chamber. A pars plana sclerectomy with a disposable MVR blade is made 3.5 mm behind the limbus. To avoid vitreous traction, an automated vitrectomy cutter without infusion is inserted until the tip is visualized through the pupil. After a small amount of vitreous is removed, viscoelastic is immediately injected through a limbal side port incision to deepen the anterior chamber.

2. Maximize visibility. With challenging cases, greater attention than usual must be paid to sharp focus, a clear tear film, and to an ocular position that optimizes the red reflex. The microscope zoom should be increased if necessary. Many techniques have been proposed for improving anterior capsule visualization in a mature white cataract. Although oblique illumination with a fiberoptic light pipe is effective, the most reliable method is the use of a dye to stain the anterior capsule.

Indocyanine green (ICG) dye, as reported by Dr. Masayuki Horiguchi[2], and trypan blue dye, as reported by Dr. Gerrit Melles[3], are both superior to fluorescein which, because it is a much smaller molecule, diffuses into the lens and vitreous. ICG (Akorn) is widely used for fundus angiography, but is not FDA approved for capsule staining. It comes as a lyophilized compound that must be mixed with 0.5 cc of diluent, and 4.5 cc of BSS Plus (Alcon, Fort Worth, Tex) immediately prior to use. Compared to trypan blue, one slight disadvantage is that larger particles often remain suspended in the ICG mixture. These appear to be eliminated during the ensuing irrigation/aspiration steps of the cataract surgery. Trypan blue dye (Vision Blue, DORC) is supplied as a premixed sterile solution. Besides the white cataract, capsular staining is helpful in other situations where the red reflex is poor, such as with a dark brunescent nucleus, or in the presence of corneal edema. An identical technique is used with either dye. The anterior chamber is filled with air to avoid excessive dilution of the dye. Several drops of dye from a TB syringe are placed through a 30-gauge cannula directly onto the anterior capsule surface, which is immediately stained. The air is then exchanged for viscoelastic, and the capsulotomy is performed in the usual manner (Figure 11-1). No special illumination is needed. The egress of white cortical "milk" may still somewhat impair visibility. In addition, if there is liquified cortex, the resulting intralenticular fluid pressure may also encourage peripheral extension of the capsular tear. Even with a capsulorrhexis, removal of the nucleus is challenging without a red reflex because the capsule edge cannot be visualized during sculpting or chopping. Dye staining of the anterior capsule is helpful in this context as well. Trypan blue dye tends to provide a more persistent staining of the capsule, which frequently lasts throughout the remainder of the procedure.

3. In higher risk eyes, the curvilinear capsular tear should be performed at a slower rate than with routine cases. To enhance control, especially in the presence of pseudoelasticity, frequently regrasp the tear to minimize the distance from the forceps to the tearing point.

4. Enlarge small pupils. When done prior to the capsulorrhexis, this improves the red reflex and provides enough working space for an adequately sized capsulotomy.

5. Since a smaller diameter capsulorrhexis is easier to control than a larger one, the former should be attempted if difficulty with visualization or control is encountered. The more peripheral the developing tear is located, the more it wants to veer centrifugally outward. This may be due to the increased convexity of the peripheral anterior capsule. In addition, a smaller capsulorrhexis increases the margin for error by allowing more opportunity to recognize and rescue a peripherally escaping tear. Once the IOL is placed, a secondary enlargement of the capsulorrhexis can be performed.

POSTERIOR CAPSULE RISK FACTORS

Conditions that increase the risk of posterior capsule rupture during phacoemulsification include ergonomic obstacles, decreased physical working space, poor visualization, increased nuclear size and density, weakened zonules, a radial tear in the capsulorrhexis, and an inability to rotate the nucleus or epinucleus.

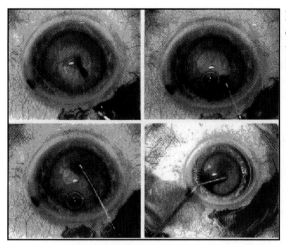

Figure 11-1. Trypan blue staining of the anterior capsule. Photo courtesy of Dutch Ophthalmic, USA, Kingston, NH.

1. Ergonomic problems make it difficult for the phaco tip to safely access the nucleus and may be either extraocular or intraocular in origin. Extraocular problems include severe esotropia, a deepset eye, a prominent brow, and an inability to position the head properly because of respiratory or musculoskeletal problems. Intraocular conditions that decrease the surgical working space include a small pupil, a small capsulorrhexis, and a shallow anterior chamber. Compared to the norm, these situations place the phaco tip closer to the iris, the capsulorrhexis, the cornea, or the posterior capsule. Excessive anterior chamber depth may result from axial myopia or a prior vitrectomy. This forces the phaco needle to approach the lens from a very steep vertical angle, which compromises both visualization and access. Sudden imbalances between fluid inflow and outflow can result from post occlusion surge, inadequate bottle height, and incisions that are too tight or too large. As more and more nucleus is removed, fluctuation in chamber depth manifests as trampolining of the posterior capsule. The amplitude of this fluctuation is exaggerated in young patients and in myopes with thin sclera because of decreased scleral rigidity.
2. Poor visualization increases the risk of cutting either the capsulorrhexis or the posterior capsule with the phaco tip. Small pupils diminish visualization in two ways. First, the peripheral lens is concealed by the iris. Second, the intensity of the red reflex is significantly reduced with each millimeter less of pupil diameter. A poor or absent red reflex makes it harder to judge the depth at which the phaco tip is cutting. Since one clue of proximity to the posterior capsule is an increasingly brighter red reflex, sculpting a deep groove is more precarious with a small pupil or a mature white lens.
3. Increased nuclear size and density elevates the risk of posterior capsule rupture. Like a pillow, a soft nucleus absorbs pressure from instrument forces. In contrast, a bulky, firm lens more resembles a stiff board in transmitting these forces directly to the posterior capsule and zonules. Maneuvers such as sculpting, rotation, and cracking all generate some lateral displacement of the nucleus, which applies stress to the capsule and the zonules. The epinucleus helps to cushion the posterior capsule against these forces. However, as the endonucleus becomes larger, the epinucleus becomes proportionately thinner, and may even be absent. Fragments generated by disassembly of a brunescent nucleus may have edges sharp enough to

puncture the capsule if sufficient pressure is applied. Finally, the deeper profile of a large endonucleus makes it difficult to completely bisect the nucleus with chopping or divide and conquer techniques. Dividing the leathery posterior plate requires one to sculpt much closer to the posterior capsule with little or no epinucleus present to shield it. Cracking it apart requires a further separation of the instrument tips which, in turn, imparts more force to the capsular bag.

4. Loose zonules pose several different problems.[4,5] First, the epinucleus and cortex do not separate as easily from a capsule that is poorly anchored. As a result, it may be difficult to rotate the nucleus, and the lax, adherent, posterior capsule may later follow the epinucleus and cortex centrally toward the aspirating instrument. Weakened zonules will dehisce more easily. Forceful sculpting or rotation of the nucleus may shear zonules in the subincisional or lateral quadrants. Aspirating the anterior capsule or adherent lens material may dehisce the zonules in that location. Stripping the cortex tangentially rather than radially helps to distribute this force upon as large an area of zonules as possible. Finally, deficient centrifugal zonular tension permits excessive trampolining of the flaccid posterior capsule during epinuclear and cortical cleanup. Redundant folds of a lax posterior capsule may be accidentally aspirated during I/A or snagged by a capsule polisher.

5. A radial tear in the capsulorrhexis can easily extend around the fornix into the posterior capsule with the application of sufficient force against the capsular bag. Such force may result from nuclear sculpting, cracking, or rotation. If a radial tear is created by the phaco tip or the second instrument, recognition may be delayed because of poor visibility during the initial stages of nuclear emulsification.

6. An inability to rotate the nucleus and epinucleus complicates any phaco technique by forcing the phaco tip to be aimed in a direction other than toward the contraincisional quadrant. Particularly with epinucleus, this increases the risk of aspirating the posterior capsule. Causes include ineffective hydrodissection, a very soft nucleus, and significant zonular laxity. As with a pillow, a soft nucleus absorbs the rotational force and is less likely to revolve as a unit. With loose zonules, the capsular bag may be so poorly fixated that it wants to rotate together with the nucleus.

STRATEGIES FOR EYES AT INCREASED RISK OF PC RUPTURE

1. Achieving a capsulorrhexis and hydrodissection are especially important when operating on a high risk eye. A capsulorrhexis renders the capsular bag more resistant to tearing. However, if the capsulorrhexis is too small, there is a greater chance that it may be incised by the phaco tip or torn by the shaft of a peripherally positioned chopper. Therefore, a wider diameter capsulorrhexis is desirable for a large, brunescent endonucleus. To maximize safety, hydrodissection should accomplish three objectives. The first goal is to be able to rotate the endonucleus with a minimum of stress applied to the zonules. The second is to be able to rotate the epinucleus. This allows the phaco tip to always aspirate the epinucleus in the contraincisional and safest quadrant. Finally, cortical cleaving hydrodissection, as described by Dr. I. Howard Fine[6], loosens the adhesion of the cortex to the capsule. The more easily the cortex separates from the capsule, the less likely it is that a floppy capsule will be pulled toward the aspirating instrument tip.

2. Surgical enlargement of the pupil should be undertaken when necessary. Besides improving surgical safety, a secondary goal is to preserve a reactive pupil of a functional size. An adequate pupil diameter is also necessary to achieve the benefits of current multifocal IOL designs. The surgical pupil size required will depend upon the surgeon's skill level and the presence of other risk factors such as exfoliation or a brunescent nucleus. Following lysis of any posterior synechiae, viscoelastic alone may expand the pupil enough for the capsulorrhexis. A maximally cohesive viscoelastic would be preferred. If the iris stroma is rigid, bimanual stretching with two lester hooks will enlarge the pupil through the creation of tiny sphincter tears.[7] This is usually the case with chronic miosis due to pilocarpine. The Beehler pupil dilator achieves this with a single instrument (Figures 11-2a and 11-2b). If the iris is floppy, the pupillary margin may simply stretch without tearing or enlarging. In this case, multiple partial-thickness sphincterotomies can be performed with Vannas or Rapazzo scissors prior to bimanual stretching. Care must be taken to avoid transecting the entire sphincter muscle. If this is still insufficient, self-retaining 5-0 nylon flexible iris retractors (Grieshaber)[8-10] may be inserted through limbal stab incisions in four quadrants to mechanically retract the iris (Figures 11-3a and 11-3b). Alternatively, an iris pupil expander ring such as the Morcher pupil dilator (Figure 11-4), or the Graether pupil expander[11] (Eagle Vision) can be used to hold the pupil open. These maneuvers should precede the capsulotomy in order to avoid hooking or tearing the capsulorrhexis margin.

3. Insertion of a Witschel endocapsular tension ring[12,13] (Morcher) is of tremendous help in the presence of zonular laxity (Figure 11-5). This can be done at any point in the procedure following completion of the requisite capsulorrhexis. Ring insertion can be accomplished using either forceps or a specially designed injector (Geuder). The PMMA tension ring partially compensates for the weakened zonular apparatus in several ways. It evenly redistributes capsular forces across all of the zonules, rather than toward a single area. The centrifugal pressure applied against the capsular fornix prevents the peripheral capsule from following the epinucleus and cortex toward the aspirating instrument tip. This pressure also keeps the posterior capsule taut, which reduces trampolining and the development of folds that can be accidentally aspirated. Postoperatively, the permanently implanted ring will resist the development of capsulophimosis, to which eyes with weak zonules are predisposed.

4. In addition to enlarging a small pupil, flexible microhook iris retractors can also be used to stabilize the capsular bag in the presence of extremely loose zonules. Self-retaining retractors are inserted through paracentesis openings in each of four quadrants to hook and fixate the capsulorrhexis. This technique of an artificial capsular support system has been reported by both Dr. Richard Mackool and Dr. Vincent Lee.[14]

5. In the presence of excessive trampolining of the posterior capsule, use of a non-coaxial separate infusion source should be considered. A self-retaining anterior chamber maintainer can be used through a limbal paracentesis either during phaco or I/A, as described by Dr. Michael Blumenthal, et al. Alternatively, a bimanual system of separate irrigation and aspiration handpieces, each introduced through snug clear corneal ports, can be helpful for epinuclear and cortical removal in these situations. In the presence of loose zonules, cortical cleanup is further facilitated by

Figure 11-2a. Beehler pupil dilator (Microtech Inc., Doylestown, Pa).

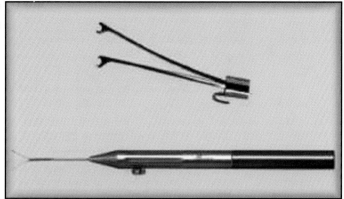

Figure 11-2b. Beehler pupil dilator.

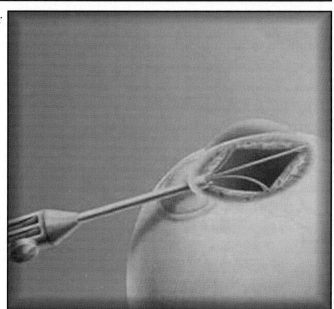

Figure 11-3a. Flexible nylon iris retractor (Grieshaber, Schaffhausen, Switzerland).

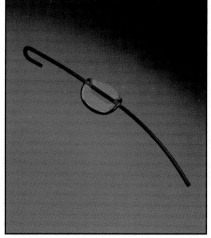

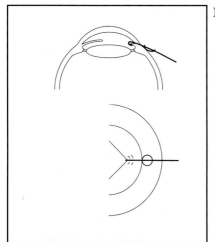

Figure 11-3b. Flexible nylon iris retractor.

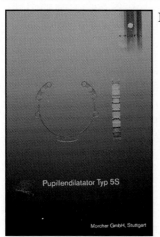

Figure 11-4. Pupil expander ring (Morcher).

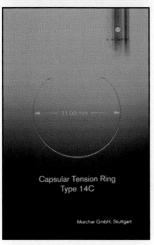

Figure 11-5. Morcher endocapsular tension ring.

the increased capsular tension provided either by an endocapsular tension ring or the haptics of the IOL. The IOL optic can block a floppy posterior capsule from reaching the I/A tip. Using a syringe and cannula, "dry" aspiration of the cortex can be accomplished using a dispersive viscoelastic to both expand the capsular fornix and restrain the lax capsule from vaulting toward the aspiration port.

PHACO TECHNIQUES FOR HIGH RISK EYES

In the presence of posterior capsule risk factors, phaco technique is a critical variable. Particular emphasis should be directed toward achieving stable chamber fluidics through the elimination of any postocclusion surge. To slow the procedure down, a lower aspiration flow rate than usual may be warranted.

It is important to employ a technique that minimizes zonular and capsular stress. The firmer and larger the nucleus, the greater the degree to which sculpting forces are transmitted to the capsular bag. To reduce movement of the nucleus during sculpting, one should sculpt at a slower rate, shave lesser amounts of nucleus with each pass, and utilize enough phaco power for the tip to cut rather than push the nucleus.

Several techniques exist that avoid intracapsular sculpting altogether and may be preferable for higher risk cases. The supracapsular flip technique, as popularized by Dr. David Brown, displaces and flips the endonucleus out of the capsular bag prior to emulsification. If accomplished, this prevents the phaco instrumentation forces from being borne by the capsular bag. Care must be taken to avoid endothelial trauma. The ease with which this flipping maneuver can be achieved varies depending upon the size of the endonucleus relative to the capsulorrhexis diameter. A nucleus that is too large or a capsulorrhexis that is too small would limit the suitability of this technique.

One of the best techniques for complicated cases is the phaco chop. Although "stop and chop" involves chopping,[15] the term "nonstop" phaco chop[16] designates pure chopping techniques that eliminate sculpting, as originally described by Dr. Kunihiro Nagahara in 1993. A Nagahara style chopper is placed peripherally beneath the anterior capsule, where it hooks the lens equator (Figure 11-6). As it moves toward the centrally impaled phaco tip, it first compresses, and then fractures the nucleus along a natural lamellar cleavage plane (Figures 11-7 and 11-8). This maneuver is repeated until nuclear fragmentation is complete (Figure 11-9).

By replacing sculpting and cracking forces with the centripetally directed manual forces of one instrument pushing against another, phaco chop reduces stress on the zonules and capsule (Figure 11-10). In sculpting, the nucleus is fixated by the capsular bag. In chopping, it is immobilized instead by the phaco tip. This significant difference in zonular stress is readily appreciated when chopping and sculpting are compared from the Miyake-Apple viewpoint in cadaver eyes.

Finally, with the elimination of sculpting, ultrasound energy is reduced[17,18] and reserved for the phaco-assisted aspiration of the individual nuclear fragments. Once these pieces have been elevated out of the capsular bag, they are emulsified at a safe distance from the posterior capsule, an advantage that phaco chop shares with other supracapsular techniques.

If hydrodissection fails, phaco chop can create the initial fragments of the nucleus without the need for sculpting or rotation. The chopper initially bisects the nucleus by moving centrally toward a stationary phaco tip. Compared to the latter, there is much

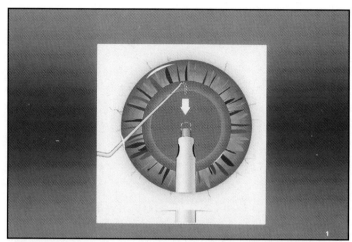

Figure 11-6. Horizontal chopper hook's equator beneath the anterior capsule.

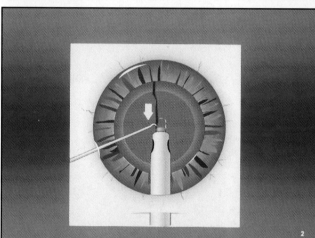

Figure 11-7. Chopper moves toward the phaco tip, compressing and fracturing the nucleus.

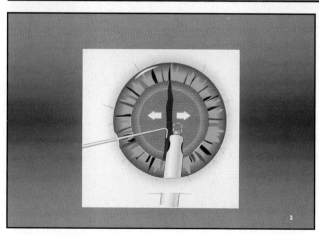

Figure 11-8. Sideways separation of the instrument tips extends the fracture through the remaining nucleus.

Figure 11-9. After slight rotation, the second chop is made.

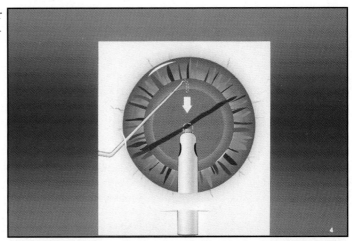

Figure 11-10. Manual instrument forces are directed centripetally inward, rather than toward the capsule and zonules.

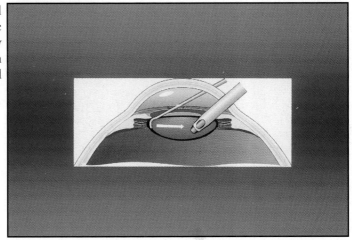

more versatility in terms of where the chopper can be placed. By repositioning the chopper several clock hours to one side, the next chop will create the first pie-shaped piece, which can then be aspirated or tumbled out.

Variations of nonstop phaco chop include Dr. Takayuki Akahoshi's prechop technique and phaco quick chop, whose originators include Drs. Hideharu Fukasaku, Abhay Vasavada,[19,20] and Vladimir Pfeiffer (Figures 11-11, 11-12, and 11-13). Although these variations all employ different strategies, they share the common advantages of reducing phaco power, phaco time, and mechanical stress on the capsule and zonules. They are therefore particularly helpful in the presence of loose zonules, a torn capsulorrhexis, and large brunescent nuclei.

SUMMARY: COMBINATION STRATEGIES

Outlining an approach for the following high-risk categories of eyes will summarize the multiple strategies that, in combination, can reduce the frequency of anterior and posterior capsule complications.

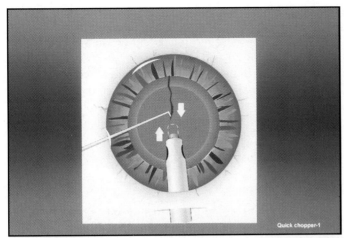

Figure 11-11. Quick chop utilizes a sharp chopper tip that penetrates the nucleus with a downward vertical motion just in front of the phaco tip.

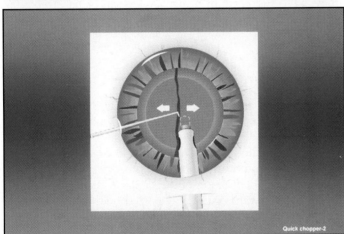

Figure 11-12. The fracture is extended with a sideways separation of the instrument tips.

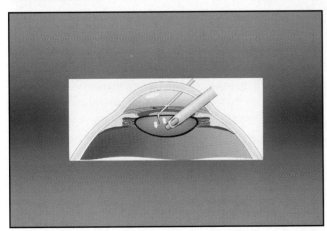

Figure 11-13. Quick chop involves a shearing force generated by movement of the instrument tips in the vertical plane.

Small Pupils

Surgically enlarging the pupil will improve the red reflex and expand the horizontal working space. This facilitates the capsulorrhexis and phacoemulsification steps. With phaco chop, the phaco tip always remains in the central 2 mm zone of the pupil where it is least likely to aspirate the iris or anterior capsule. Because it is a kinesthetic technique that, unlike sculpting, does not require visualization of the depth of the phaco tip, there is less dependence upon a bright red reflex. Supracapsular flipping techniques can bring the nucleus into the pupillary plane so that the emulsification takes place just anterior to the pupil. Iris retractors or a pupil expander ring may be needed for a floppy, elastic iris.

Narrow Angles/Shallow AC

The most cohesive viscoelastics may be required to deepen the AC for the capsulorrhexis. Phaco chop, by reducing phaco power and time, may be a safer technique because of the closer proximity of the endothelium. A mechanical pars plana vitreous tap can convert a flat chamber to one of normal depth. This creates enough clearance to enlarge the pupil, complete a capsulorrhexis, and phaco the nucleus at a safer distance from the endothelium.

Mature Cataracts (White or Brown)

ICG or trypan blue dye provides excellent visualization of the anterior capsule both during the capsulotomy and during phaco. In the presence of high intralenticular fluid pressure, the capsulorrhexis should be made smaller. If the nucleus is large and brunescent, phaco chop can reduce stress on the zonules and decrease overall phaco time. Although the red reflex is poor or absent, phaco chop is a more kinesthetic maneuver and, unlike sculpting, does not require visualization of the depth of the phaco tip. If a can opener capsulotomy is necessary, outward cracking motions should be minimized in favor of inwardly directed chopping maneuvers.

Loose Zonules

To improve control of a pseudoelastic capsule, a small diameter capsulotomy coupled with frequent regrasping of the flap may be necessary. An endocapsular tension ring more evenly distributes instrument forces across all of the zonules. It can also reduce the tendency for a lax posterior capsule to trampoline forward. Flexible iris retractors can immobilize an otherwise unstable capsule. Phaco chop minimizes stress placed upon the capsule by using centripetally directed, opposing instrument forces to segment the endonucleus.

REFERENCES

1. Gimbel HV, Neuhann T. Development, advantages, and methods of the continuous circular capsulorrhexis technique. *J Cataract Refract Surg*. 1990;16:31-37.
2. Horiguchi M, Miyake K, Ohta I, Ito Y. Staining of the lens capsule for circular continuous capsulorrhexis in eyes with white cataract. *Arch Ophthalmol*. 1998;116:535-537.
3. Melles G, de Waard P, Pameyer J, Beekhuis W. Trypan blue capsule staining to visualize the capsulorrhexis in cataract surgery. *J Cataract Refract Surg*. 1999;25:7-9.

4. Osher RH, Cionni RJ, Gimbel HV, Crandall AS. Cataract surgery in patients with pseudoexfoliation syndrome. *Eur J Implant Ref Surg*. 1993;5:46-50.

5. Fine IH, Hoffman RS. Phacoemulsification in the presence of pseudoexfoliation: challenges and options. *J Cataract Refract Surg*. 1997;23:160-165.

6. Fine IH. Cortical cleaving hydrodissection. *J Cataract Refract Surg*. 1992;18:508-512.

7. Miller KM, Keener GT Jr. Stretch pupillpolasty for small pupil phacoemulsification. *Am J Ophthalmol*. 1994;117:107-108.

8. De Juan E, Hickingbotham D. Flexible iris retractor (letter). *Am J Ophthalmol*. 1991;111: 776-777.

9. Nichamin LD. Enlarging the pupil for cataract extraction using flexible nylon iris retractors. *J Cataract Refract Surg*. 1993;19:793-796.

10. Masket S. Avoiding complications associated with iris retractor use in small pupil cataract extraction. *J Cataract Refract Surg*. 1996;22:168-171.

11. Graether JM. Graether pupil expander for managing the small pupil during surgery. *J Cataract Refract Surg*. 1996;22:530-535.

12. Witschel BM, Legler U. New approaches to zonular cases; the capsular ring. *Audiovisual J Cataract Implant Surg*. 1993;9(4).

13. Masket S, ed. Consultation section. *J Cataract Refract Surg*. 1998;24:1289-1298.

14. Lee V, Bloom P. Microhook capsule stabilization for phacoemulsification in eyes with pseudoexfoliation-syndrome-induced lens instability. *J Cataract Refract Surg*. 1999;25:1567-1570.

15. Koch PS, Katzen LE. Stop and chop phacoemulsification. *J Cataract Refract Surg*. 1994;20:566-570.

16. Chang D. Converting to phaco chop: Why? Which technique? How? *Ophthalmic Practice*. 1999;17(4):202-210.

17. DeBry P, Olson RJ, Crandall AS. Comparison of energy required for phaco-chop and divide and conquer phacoemulsification. *J Cataract Refract Surg*. 1998;24:689-692.

18. Ram J, Wesendahl TA, Auffarth GU, Apple DJ. Evaluation of in situ fracture versus phaco chop techniques. *J Cataract Refract Surg*. 1998;24:1464-1468.

19. Vasavada AR, Desai, JP. Stop, chop, chop and stuff. *J Cataract Refract Surg*. 1996;22:526-529.

20. Vasavada A, Singh R. Step-by-step chop in situ and separation of very dense cataracts. *J Cataract Refract Surg*. 1998;24:156-159.

12 Intraocular Lens Design and Materials

Randall J. Olson, MD

INTRODUCTION

The transition to foldable intraocular lenses was forced by phacoemulsification (phaco). Issues such as posterior capsular opacification (PCO), biocompatibility, and any of the other issues that will be discussed simply were not considerations in moving toward foldable lenses. After all, polymethylmethacrylate (PMMA) intraocular lenses (IOLs) were the gold standard, so who needed anything more? The early driving force for foldables was simply to keep the phaco wound intact. Very few realized that Kelman's phaco would create a demand for new designs, just as capsulorrhexis guaranteed dependable bag fixation. The first materials to rise to the challenge were hydrogel and first-generation silicone.

Hydrogels have always suffered from the problem of fragility and would not hold up to the pressure of being pushed through a small wound.[1] Therefore, the first clinically accepted foldable material was first-generation silicone, which developed a small but growing group of adherents that were required to enlarge the wound slightly, taking the wound from 6.0 mm or more in size down to about 4.0 mm. The early days of silicone IOLs, however, were rocky with yttrium-aluminum-garnet laser (YAG) capsulotomy found to be more difficult, resulting in more noticeable YAG damage.[2] Then, there was the report of yellowing with the prediction by some alarmists that silicone IOLs of today would be the cataracts of tomorrow (Figure 12-1).[3] There were reports of increased inflammation, yet the technique advantage won out in the end. By altering how we approach laser capsulotomy, as well as manufacturing process improvements, the capsulotomy and yellowing issues have disappeared, and most of these IOLs are doing just fine.

Plate IOLs were the pioneering design, and they lent themselves to insertion devices that allowed full advantage of the small incision. PMMA adherents did not want to be left out of the race, so we saw a move to oval and sub 6.0 mm optic IOLs. The oval IOL suffered from increased dysphotopsia[4] and has been virtually eliminated from the market. The 5.5 mm round PMMA IOL, however, became well accepted as a good compromise and is still commonly used today.

Figure 12-1. Slit lamp photo of severe silicone IOL haze. This represents water in the periphery of the silicone material. Fortunately this problem has been resolved with technological advances.

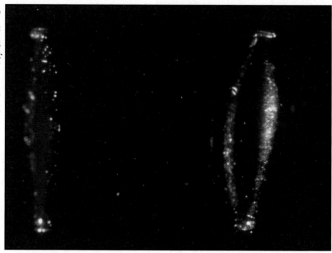

FOLDING IOLs: THE SMALL INCISION ADVANTAGE

In 1992, in the midst of all of these changes, Alan Crandall and I surveyed the field and felt that foldable IOLs would be important for the future. SLM2 silicone (Allergan SI-30, Allergan Medical Optics, Irvine, Calif) had just been released and had some interesting features including, as a second-generation silicone, an increased refractive index for a much thinner profile with a lenticular design promoting constant center thickness. It had good ultraviolet (UV) filtration that was not available in plate silicone at the time, and therefore, we felt that a head-to-head comparison between the SI-30 IOL and a 5.5 mm round PMMA IOL in a long-term masked prospective trial could answer some important questions raised by the naysayers in regard to foldable lenses. Certainly, everyone accepted that there may be some short-term advantages; however, there was no study showing that, long-term, it really made any difference which lens was used. We both felt comfortable with a superior scleral tunnel incision and sutureless wounds for both the 5.5 PMMA and the SI-30, so that our comparison was totally based on incision size and not our surgical technique. We were comfortable with a randomized schedule in that we did not necessarily know which lens would be better long-term.

We enrolled 119 patients with uncomplicated surgery, without the need for sutures in either group. Our original analysis is still the easiest to understand and uses with-the-rule astigmatism change as plus and against-the-rule as minus for this 12 o'clock incision. We analyzed astigmatism, LogMAR visual acuity with and without correction, and percent astigmatism shifts over 1 D, all of which showed a 3-year postoperative statistically significant advantage in favor of the smaller incision (Table 12-1). After completion of this study,[5] we were confident that patients are better off with foldable IOLs. The market has certainly responded, with foldable lenses already representing the majority of those used, and this trend is increasing.[6]

IOLs AND INCIDENCE OF PCO

The one big surprise in this entire study was the visual acuity difference with correction. If the only impact was a wound effect, then how could best-corrected vision differ

Table 12-1

Postoperative Astigmatism

	Day 1	Day 8	Day 30	3 Months	6 Months	1 Years	3 Years	3 Years Vision Without Correction	3 Years With Correction
Number	110	117	114	99	82	85	84	59**	59**
3.2 mm	0.11	0.11	0.13	-0.02	-0.02	-0.07	-0.13	0.15**	0.07**
5.5 mm	-0.22	-0.41	-0.37	-0.50	-0.55	-0.55	-0.75	0.26**	0.12**
P*	0.03	0.0001	0.0001	0.0001	0.0001	0.0001	0.0001	0.03**	0.05**

Measurements of astigmatism are in diopters

*by student's *t* test

**LogMAR vision; best case analysis (20/20=0.00)

between the two lens groups? This prompted a more complete PCO review of patients with both an objective and subjective means of scoring these differences. For our objective measuring device, we use the lens opacity meter, which quantitatively measures reflected light and was intended as a tool to evaluate cataract progression. We also had a slit lamp evaluation system as our subjective measure, both of which were done in a masked fashion. What we found in both analyses was a statistically significant decrease in PCO in comparison to PMMA (Table 12-2).[7] Such a conclusion had not been suggested for silicone, and we were further intrigued with the concept that PCO is more than just a YAG capsulotomy concern (retinal detachment and cost), but also has an impact on our patient's vision prior to capsulotomy. We often forget that many patients do not necessarily come back to have their capsules opened in a timely fashion and that in many areas of the country, patients have to drop quite significantly in vision before a capsulotomy is allowed. This is a real quality of life concern in trying to avoid PCO.

When it comes to prevention of PCO, the lens that usually comes to mind is the Alcon AcrySof (Alcon Surgical, Fort Worth, Tex) series of IOLs. We were very interested in what a head-to-head comparison between SLM2 silicone and AcrySof might look like at the completion of our study, because when we first set up our protocol, AcrySof was not clinically available. Fortunately, in December 1998,[8] Hayashi reported such a study with a comparison of PMMA, AcrySof, and the SI-30 IOL in a prospective, randomized, long-term (2-year) clinical trial. They looked at their YAG capsulotomy rates, as well as objectively measuring PCO using Scheimpflug photography. What they found was a statistically significant advantage of both the SI-30 (SLM2 silicone) and AcrySof over PMMA in regard to YAG capsulotomy rates, objective scores of PCO, and visual acuity with correction. Interestingly, the results between AcrySof and SLM2 silicone were similar and not statistically different for all three parameters. This study confirmed our finding in regard to the differences between SLM2 silicone and PMMA, PCO and visual acuity. Now we had documentation of two IOL styles that can make a major difference in regard to PCO. The FDA has responded by allowing a claim for PCO prevention for PhacoFlex II SLM2 silicone by Allergan.

Table 12-2

Three-year Results Relating to Posterior Capsular Opacification (N=84)

	Rate of YAG Laser Capsulotomy	Percentage of Reflected Light*	PCO Score**
Silicone IOL	24%	8.6%	0.882
PMMA IOL	33%	10.4%	1.792

PCO = posterior capsular opacification; IOL = intraocular lens;

PMMA = polymethylmethacrylate

*Tested by light opacity meter (P = .02, student's t-test)

** Scale of subjective scoring: 0-4+, where 0 represents no opacity and 4+ represents dense posterior capsule opacification. (P = .0001, Student's t-test).

Adapted from: Olson RJ, Crandall AS. Silicone versus polymethylmethacrylate intraocular lenses with regard to capsular opacification. *Ophthalmic Surg Lasers.* 1998;29:57.

The story is not complete, however, without discussing a more recent paper by Hollick, et al,[10] which was also a prospective randomized head-to-head comparison between AcrySof, silicone, and PMMA. They used retroillumination photographs as a means of measuring PCO and found AcrySof again distinctly superior to PMMA; however, silicone in this instance was, if anything, only slightly better than PMMA. This well done and interesting study, however, used first generation silicone, supporting the earlier anecdotal statements that silicone did not have any PCO advantage and also clearly showed that all silicone is not alike. Just as we are going to have to differentiate between the different acrylic IOLs, this shows we must differentiate between silicone materials with, at this point in time at least, SLM2 silicone being the only one shown to have a PCO advantage (Table 12-3).

It is a major advantage for our patients to be able to inhibit PCO. However, neither AcrySof nor SLM2 silicone was developed as a means of PCO prevention. So, how do they work? Nishi has reported and published information about biomechanical factors in PCO prevention and has shown that a discontinuous bend in the posterior capsule is an important factor.[11] AcrySof's squared edge clearly produces such a discontinuous bend; in fact, Nishi has reported that he can duplicate the AcrySof effect in rabbits with a PMMA lens that has a similar squared off edge (Figure 12-2).[12] At a symposium at ESCRS 1999, he further reported some prevention using a flattened edge silicone IOL and a loss of PCO prevention when he rounded the edge of AcrySof.[13] Although AcrySof capsular tackiness was thought to be a factor, at this point in time it would appear that AcrySof PCO prevention is due to this flattened edge creating a discontinuous bend in the capsule.

Due to the fact that all of the SLM2 silicone IOLs currently used have rounded edges, other biomaterial effects must be important in regard to PCO prevention. One factor to consider is hydrophilicity, or the lack thereof, and its impact on lens epithelial cell growth. Two recent studies,[14,15] one in vitro and one clinical, have shown that increased hydrophilicity clearly encourages[16] lens epithelial cell growth. The clinical article by

Table 12-3

Comparison of Capsular Opacification With Different Lens Styles

Study	IOL Type	Postop Follow-up	PCO*	% with Laser Capsulotomy	% No Loss of Visual Acuity**
Hayashi, et al‡	PMMA Allergan	2 years	26	30%	25%
	SI-30 NB (silicone) Alcon MA-60BM	2 years	12	6%	73%
	AcrySof	2 years	16	3%	73%
	P-value SI-30 and AcrySof vs. PMMA		< .001	< .001	< .001
Hollick, et al§	PMMA	3 years	56%	26%	N/A
	Lolab L141U first-generation silicone	3 years	40%	14%	N/A
	Alcon MA-60 BM, AcrySof	3 years	10%	0%	N/A
	P-Value MA-60 vs. L141U + PMMA		< .001	0.05	

*Represents posterior capsular opacification measured objectively by Schiempflug photography in the Hayashi study and by retroillumination photographs in the Hollick study.

**Loss of vision at end of the study best corrected compared to best corrected postoperative vision.

‡Adapted from: Hayashi H, Hayashi K, Nakao F, Hayashi F. Quantitative comparison of posterior capsule opacification after polymethylmethacrylate, silicone, and soft acrylic intraocular lens implantation. *Arch Ophthalmol*. 1998; 116:1579-1582.

§Adapted from: Hollick EJ, Spalton DJ, Ursell PG, et al. The effect of polymethylmethacrylate, silicone, and polyacrylic intraocular lenses on posterior capsular opacification 3 years after cataract surgery. *Ophthalmology*. 1999; 106:49-54.

Hollick, et al shows an inverse relationship between lens epithelial growth and inflammation, in that patients with a hydrophilic acrylic IOL with minimal inflammation seemed to correlate well with increased lens epithelial cell growth on the anterior surface. On the other hand, hydrophobicity did not allow lens epithelial cell growth, which may be a factor in the prevention of PCO. The Hollick study suggested that hydrophilic acrylics as a group may have a problem with PCO; it cited one study report by their group in a clinical trial that suggested exactly that. At this point in time, it is too soon to say whether PCO will be a problem for hydrophilic acrylics; however, it appears unlikely they will have a PCO advantage from a biomaterials standpoint. Good prospective, randomized trials will be important to either validate or refute this supposition. Will a flattened-edge hydrophilic acrylic lens with its biomechanical effect more than compensate

Figure 12-2. A squared-edge PMMA IOL creates a discontinuous bend in the capsule with similar PCO prevention to AcrySof. (Reprinted from: Nishi O, Nishi K. Preventing posterior capsule opacification by creating a discontinuous sharp bend in the capsule. *J Cataract Refract Surg.* 1999;25(4):521-526.)

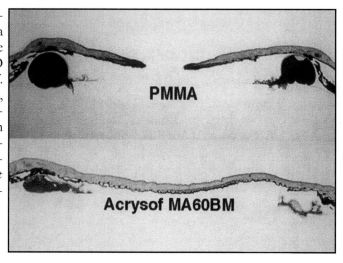

for a possible biomaterials disadvantage? Does SLM2 silicone with a flattened edge have both a biomaterial and a biomechanical effect? Such are the exciting questions that we can pose as we look at changes in material that I feel are inevitable. What I would really like to see is a full understanding of the biomaterial advantage of SLM2 silicone in that it cannot just be hydrophobicity. This material is no more hydrophobic than other silicone material, and yet there is a difference in PCO advantage between SLM2 silicone and first generation silicones. As we understand these effects and use them in new products we will gain an even greater PCO edge.

The PCO story is not complete without discussing the potential downside to a flattened edge. AcrySof is an interesting material with a very high refractive index that can cause a cosmetically objectionable pupil reflection. This is generally a minor annoyance; however, it has been a cause for explantation to a few patients.[16] Other than this cosmetic reflection, I certainly did not feel there were other dysphotopsia issues until a peace officer came to see me with complaints of disabling night reflections that made it impossible for him to work at night. He talked about central flashes of light, no matter where he tried to look at oncoming headlights, as absolutely disabling. On examination, I found a perfectly centered MA30 (5.5 mm optic) AcrySof lens with the capsule over the edge of the IOL for 360 degrees. There was no PCO and the patient was 20/15 uncorrected. He had already seen multiple ophthalmologists who told him that there was nothing wrong and simply had written him off as crazy. He was desperate for relief, and I found him a very believable historian.

After talking to a colleague who had a similar case resolved after IOL exchange, we decided, with careful informed consent, to remove this seemingly perfect result and replace it with an SI40 IOL. The patient reported relief in the recovery room, and on the first postoperative day stated he had complete resolution of his symptoms. This dysphotopsia is an unintended consequence of the flattened edge of AcrySof, and we have reported on eight patients with nine operated eyes between our group and Jules Stein Institute who required IOL exchange for relief of their symptoms.[17] The majority of these patients had large pupils at night and had a 5.5 mm optic; however, this also occurred in patients with a 6.0 mm optic. All were insistent upon something being done about their symptoms and had either complete or substantial relief of their symptoms with any round edge IOL. As we pursue an ongoing survey of explanted lenses at our institution, sponsored by the American Society of Cataract and Refractive Surgery, indeed we see a distinct difference in foldable IOLs for the reasons of explantation. The number one reason for explantation of the AcrySof lenses has been unwanted images, while for three-piece silicone it has been incorrect IOL power, and for plate lenses it has been dislocation. The other IOL in which removal for dysphotopsia can occur is the Array multifocal intraocular lens. The Array can produce unwanted night images, which is a natural physical result of the different refractive zones on the lens. While engineering around this problem with night vision for multifocal lenses would seem to be difficult, getting around the problem with the flattened edge seems to me to be a simpler engineering problem.

Holladay[18] has documented exactly what is happening using ray tracing analysis. The flattened edge in AcrySof acts like a mirror such that off-centered lights can cause a central flash, which is what patients have reported (Figure 12-3). Although we found pilocarpine can be helpful, it usually does not sufficiently alleviate the symptoms in those who are severely bothered. Opacification of the capsule over the edge of the AcrySof would also solve the problem; however, just as it prevents PCO, AcrySof is also very successful for the same reason in preventing anterior capsular opacification;[19] therefore, this remedy generally does not work. We need the PCO advantage of the flattened edge without this dysphotopsia concern and look forward to the optical and manufacturing engineers to figure out how to provide this.

This has real impact in regard to overall patient outcomes and their perceptions of difficulties, in particular with night driving. In a recent outcomes analysis of postoperative cataract patients,[20] we found the SI40 IOL performed better than all other IOLs studied in regard to night driving vision. As already mentioned, many patients experienced night dysphotopsia symptoms with the MA30 and MA60 IOL. Interestingly, some normal controls and SI40 patients also complained a lot.[14] Understanding dysphotopsia and working on means to alleviate the symptoms is an important area for us as we improve the quality of our outcomes from the present level of excellence to an even higher level of acceptance.

A new dysphotopsia syndrome unique to AcrySof was recently reported by Davison.[21] He described this as idiopathic temporal darkness that is seen as a graying or graininess of temporal vision, which can be so severe that explantation is the only solution. While this symptom usually gets better with time, Dr. Davison reported six patients out of 800 who complained, and three that will be explanted. This concern is so new that I have little to add to the feeling that the flattened edge and high refractive index must be involved. Is this some complex nasal shadow? I am sure we will hear more about this phenomenon.

GLISTENINGS IN ACRYLIC OPTIC

There was a lot of excitement when AcrySof was first released as a new foldable material in the United States. We implanted many AcrySof IOLs and were amazed that in 2 to 3 weeks, we had a large group of our patients with multiple inclusions (Figure 12-4), in some cases appearing almost as a confluent and profound whitening of the lens. This was totally unexpected and something we immediately reported.[22] Fortunately, we had a small cohort of uncomplicated patients with a silicone IOL in one eye and an AcrySof IOL with glistenings in the second eye for comparison. Our numbers were very small;

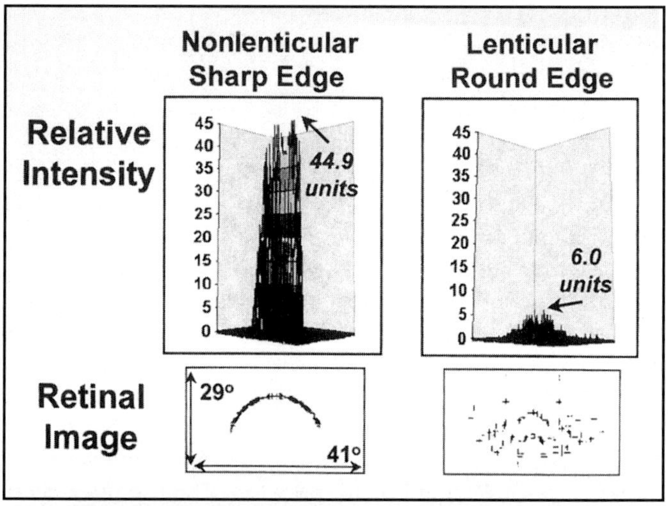

Figure 12-3. Ray tracing analysis shows the round edge of an IOL disperses a peripheral light source, while a flattened edge can create a "mirror-like" effect bouncing the image into the central vision. (Reprinted from: Holladay JT, Lange A, Portney V. Analysis of edge glare phenomena intraocular lens edge designs. *J Cataract Refract Surg.* 1999;750.)

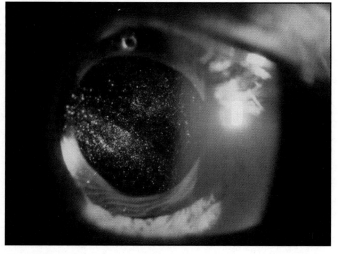

Figure 12-4. A slit lamp photograph of a patient with many "glistenings" (water vacuoles) in an AcrySof intraocular lens. (Reprinted from: Dhaliwal OK, Mamalis N, Olson RJ, et al. Visual significance of glistenings seen in the AcrySof IOL. *J Cataract Refract Surg.* 1996;22:452-457.)

however, we did find a statistically significant loss of contrast sensitivity in association with these glistenings, and we felt this was a clinical issue of some concern.

AcrySof IOLs were temporarily removed from the marketplace and it was determined that these glistenings were small vacuoles of water scattered throughout the IOL, which when unusually large result in this clinical appearance. These inclusions were very easy to duplicate in the laboratory, and we were able to determine that there was something different about the micro environment of the lens when sterilized in the Acrypak holder (Alcon Laboratories, Fort Worth, Tex), in comparison to the previous wagon wheel packaging that had been used.[23] These acute glistenings were only found in the Acrypak system. Fortunately, we found these acute glistenings became better with time and with a change to the wagon wheel configuration, this issue appeared to be resolved.

Although there had been concerns raised since then about these inclusions with the AcrySof IOL, it was a poster by Mitooka at the 1999 ASCRS annual meeting[24] that again raised the issue for me. This report on late-onset glistenings concluded the problem was more severe with diabetes, unexplained visual loss in two patients, and a net overall loss of contrast sensitivity comparing minimal and no glistenings to those with significant glistenings. We had also noted late-onset glistenings along with some that appeared as severe as our first report, and so commenced our own new study.

We looked only at wagon wheel AcrySof lenses that had not shown the acute glistenings we had previously reported. We used a random selection process over time to look at 42 patients for intensive study and review of this phenomenon. We found four patients with a grade of three to four plus glistenings, which is defined as 30 or more glistenings in a slit beam set at 10 x 2 mm. Further studies showed a mean visual acuity of those at two plus or less glistening of 20/22.1 versus 20/25.5, for more severe glistenings, which was statistically significant (P=0.01). Evaluations for whether this was progressive over time were strongly suggestive (P=0.085) with the majority of patients, with trace glistenings being those less than 1 year postoperative (Table 12-4).[25]

The whole subject of AcrySof glistenings is poorly understood. The evidence at this time would suggest that there is the potential for some contrast and minor visual acuity loss, especially in diabetics. How much this might be progressive with time and whether greater clinical significance might occur is certainly unclear; however, this deserves more complete studies than either Mitooka or ours. Clearly, chronic glistenings are an area of some concern and deserve further evaluation.

Biocompatibility has been excellent for all available foldable materials. However, differences among the materials are certainly becoming evident. In a recent Hollick study already quoted,[14] the Hydroview lens, a hydrophilic acrylic, was better than PMMA and SLM2 silicone for small-cell inflammatory adhesions; however, SLM2 silicone and Hydroview were equal and both much better than PMMA in regard to the more clinically important giant cell deposits. In another study,[26] the same group showed that first generation silicone was more like PMMA, and that both were worse than AcrySof when looking at giant cell deposits. Ravalico[27] showed SLM2 silicone and hydrophilic acrylic to be equal, with both being better than heparin surface-modified PMMA, all of which were much better than PMMA in regard to giant cell deposits (See Table 12-3).

Samuelson, a glaucoma surgeon, was concerned about giant cell deposits in phaco and IOL combined with trabeculectomy. These high-risk patients, often with chronic pilocarpine use requiring pupil stretch, can have significant giant cell deposits that can impede vision and, therefore, which lens style would be the safest to implant was an important issue for study. He entered into a prospective, randomized study looking at 6-month postoperative results comparing SLM2 silicone (Allergan SI-30 and 40), first generation silicone plate lenses (C10 and C11), and AcrySof. Interestingly, he found that the SLM2 silicone performed statistically better than first-generation silicone. SLM2 silicone showed a 5% incidence of deposits, while first-generation silicone was significantly worse with 33%. AcrySof was in the middle with about 15% having giant cell deposits.[28] Again, we now have multiple studies confirming that silicone material must be differentiated, and at least SLM2 silicone (Allergan SI-30, 40, 55, and Array) is clinically different in regard to biocompatibility over first-generation silicone (Table 12-5).

One interesting attribute of the hydrophilic acrylic memory lens is that in its rolled dehydrated state, it substantially blocks light when first inserted. Unless someone waits until the lens is fully hydrated and unrolled, which takes many minutes, this could be protective of operating microscope-induced retinal phototoxicity. In a study we did using an optical bench, it would appear that this light blockage effect is indeed quite profound early on and that during the clinical time frame of surgery this should be a clinical advan-

Table 12-4

A 4-Year Study of Chronic Water Vacuoles (Glistenings) in Alcon AcrySof Intraocular Lenses

- 5 of 42 (12%) rated 3-4+
- 14 of 15 (93%) found greater than trace glistenings had been implanted for longer than 1 year (P=.085)
- Snellen best-corrected visual acuity was 20/22.1 for those less than 2+ glistenings; 20/25.5 for those with 2+ or greater glistenings (P=.01)

Adapted from: Christiansen G, Durcan FJ, Olson RJ, Christiansen K. Prevalence, severity, and visual significance of glistenings seen in the AcrySof IOLs one to four years from implantation. *J Cataract Refract Surg*. In press.

tage. We also found that determining the actual power of the IOL was very difficult. IOL power accuracy will be more difficult to control with hydrophilic acrylics. Whether this is a clinical problem remains to be seen.[29]

SURFACE MODIFICATION

Heparin surface modification is the first clinically-accepted coated IOL. This concept dates back to the early days of specular microscopy in the previscoelastic era, when IOLs were shown to potentially create corneal endothelial damage.[30] Any contact between the IOL and the corneal endothelium could be devastating. It was also well-known in the early days that if the IOL was coated with a hydrophilic substance, a surgeon could block the contact damage between the lens and the endothelium.[31] We were able to verify this with IOLs coated with a hydrophilic substance in a cat study that was never published in preparation for human clinical trial. The rest of this story is interesting in that unusual inflammation in the clinical trial, probably secondary to heat-stable endotoxin, resulted in such severe uveitis that there was some loss of vision and the study was cancelled.[32] With the era of closed intraocular surgery using viscoelastic, the issue became moot.

The concept of surface modification of IOLs did not die in the viscoelastic era. A method of enhancing the biocompatibility of a PMMA IOL called surface passivation later received mixed reviews and never became clinically important. Heparin surface-modified PMMA has been accepted clinically as being more biocompatible than regular PMMA.[33,34] Some feel this is the lens of choice in uveitis patients. However, as mentioned above, some foldables such as SLM2 silicone and hydrophilic acrylic may actually be better than heparin-surfaced modified lenses in some of these high risk cases.[26,14,29,27] There is still a lot more to be done in this area. I foresee an era in which the anterior surface of an IOL may be coated for increased hydrophilicity, and the posterior surface coated in a way to decrease PCO. A surface coating toxic to lens epithelial cells has also been discussed; therefore, I think the concept of coating lenses is still an important one, and that we will see breakthroughs in the future. What can be said at this time is that we clearly have lens groups that are superior to PMMA in regard to biocom-

Table 12-5

Comparison of Giant Cell Deposits on Different Lens Materials

Study	IOL	Postop Time	% Deposits
Ravalico*	PMMA	6 months	60%
(routine surgery)	Pharmacia HSM PMMA	6 months	10%
	Alcon Logel	6 months	0
	Allergan SI-30NB silicone	6 months	0
Hollick†	PMMA	2 years	Maximum 40%
(routine surgery)	Iolab L141U First-generation silicone	2 years	Maximum 33%
	Alcon MA60	2 years	0
			$P = .003$
Hollick‡	PMMA	2 years, 6 months	27%
	Allergan SI 30 Second-generation silicone	6 months	0
	Storz H60M Hydroview	6 months	2
			$P < .001$
Samuelson§ (phaco, IOL, and trabeculectomy)	Allergan SI-30 40 second-generation silicone	6 months	5%
	Starr C10/C11 First-generation silicone	6 months	33%
	Alcon MA 60 BM AcrySof	6 months	15%
			$P < .001$

*Adapted from: Ravalico G, Baccara F, Lovisato A, Tognetto D. Postoperative cellular reaction on various intraocular lens materials. *Ophthalmology*. 1997;104:1084-1091.

†Adapted from: Hollick EJ, Spalton DJ, Ursell PG, Pande MV. Biocompatibility of polymethyl methacrylate, silicone, and AcrySof intraocular lenses: randomized comparison of the cellular reaction on the anterior lens surface. *J Cataract Refract Surg*. 1998;24:361-366.

‡Adapted from: Hollick EJ, Spalton DJ, Ursell PG. Surface cytologic features on intraocular lenses: can increased biocompatibility have disadvantages? *Arch Ophthalmol*. 1999;117:872-878.

§Adapted from: Samuelson TW, Chu YR,Kreiger RA. Prospective randomized evaluation of giant cell deposits on foldable IOLs following combined cataract and glaucoma surgery. *J Cataract Refract Surg*. 2000;26:817-823.

patibility. These include AcrySof, heparin surfaced-modified PMMA, hydrophilic acrylic, and SLM2 silicone. Getting the perfect match between biocompatibility and PCO inhibition is where the exciting advances will be seen in the future.

FOLDABLE IOLs AND INCISION SIZE

The whole field of foldable IOLs started because of wound size, yet we have a large disparity in wound size among the different foldables. Memmen,[35] at the Hawaii Eye Meeting 1999 using Deacon-Steinart gauges (Capital Instruments Ltd., Wan Chai, Hong Kong), found a range of final incision sizes from 2.65 mm for the SI55 with the Unfolder system, up to 3.9 mm for the MA-60 AcrySof inserted with forceps. We were able to prove that going from an approximately 5.5 mm size to a 3.2 mm size was clinically and statistically significant.[5] However, is going from a sub 3.0 mm to a 4.0 mm final wound size of any clinical importance? Certainly this deserves another careful, controlled, prospective clinical trial to see. Indeed, what happens to long-term astigmatism with variations of sub 3.0 to 4.0 mm wound sizes? However, such a study would likely be a long and arduous task, and to my knowledge no such studies have been entered into at this time. One item we felt we could look at, however, is the very real issue of wound complications created at the time of surgery. There are lenses that can easily be inserted without increasing the size of the wound after phacoemulsification, with other lenses clearly requiring enlargement of the wound. There are approximately 4000 surgical procedures done annually at the Moran Eye Center with a mixture of faculty, fellows, and residents performing these surgeries. The two most popular lenses are AcrySof and SI-40; a head-to-head comparison of wound complications with similar optic size between the MA-60 AcrySof with a mean final wound size of approximately 3.9 mm versus the SI-40 with the Unfolder with a mean wound size of approximately 3.0 mm would at least answer the wound complication issue.

We looked at 200 consecutive uncomplicated cases in which either the MA-60 AcrySof or the SI-40 intraocular lens was used. These were all topical and temporal sutureless incisions with the Unfolder used for the SI-40 without wound enlargement, and the wound enlarged in all instances for the AcrySof IOL inserted with insertion forceps.

We specifically looked in the operative report for the need for placement of sutures due to a leaky wound and/or a leaky wound on the first postoperative day. We found 13 such wound events out of 200 cases for the AcrySof IOL, and three such wound events for the SI-40 IOL. This difference was statistically significant (P=0.01). At our institution, we concluded that wound enlargement in topical, sutureless, clear corneal surgery does create a more unstable wound. All else being equal, this is best avoided.[16] The question of long-term stability of astigmatism and uncorrected visual acuity still deserves to be studied.

SILICONE IOLs AND SILICONE OIL

Another issue with silicone IOLs is the use of silicone oil for complicated retinal detachments with coating of the posterior silicone lens surface if the capsule is open, resulting in markedly decreased visualization of the fundus. This is a problem that exists as well for PMMA and AcrySof, but less so than silicone. Hydrophilic acrylics appear to have a distinct advantage in regard to this issue. The visualization problem has been reported to be severe enough that removal of the IOL may be necessary at the time of posterior segment work with silicone oil or for visualization of the posterior segment after silicone oil use.[36]

While silicone oil use is overall an event in a very small percentage of patients, the concern is about silicone ever being used in a patient who is at any risk for complicated vitreoretinal pathology. Recently, a German group[37] reported a solvent that immediately cleared all IOLs in contact with silicone oil for perfect visualization (Figures 12-5a and 12-5b). While clinical studies regarding biocompatibility of this material have not been done, its chemical makeup would appear likely to make it acceptable; therefore, with time I expect this to be another example of an issue that will be resolved by technology. Similarly, I feel that the crystalline inclusions in AcrySof IOLs will eventually be understood and, with a change in material, will be resolved. For instance, the Allergan Sensar acrylic IOL, which is approved in Europe, does not have inclusion concerns, appears to be less brittle and more easily folded, and can be used with an insertion device that allows a significantly smaller wound size than AcrySof. We should continue to expect improvement in materials and resolution of the clinical concerns of today through development and competition.[37]

SUMMARY

What conclusions can be drawn from this remarkable field of success that represents our world of IOL use today?

1. It is clear that the future is the foldable IOL with real advantages in regard to wound stability with better long-term astigmatism and visual acuity results that make for an easier surgical procedure and better outcomes for our patients.

2. We now have materials that provide clear PCO advantage over PMMA. This translates into decreased need for optical capsulotomy and better long-term corrected vision for our patients. PCO prevention appears to be both a biomechanical (the flattened edge of Alcon AcrySof for a barrier effect) and a biomaterial (Allergan Phacoflex II) effect. At this time, Allergan Phacoflex II SLM2 silicone and Alcon AcrySof have demonstrated a PCO advantage that appears to be about equal. Hydrophilic acrylics, without any optic edge manipulation, will probably have a PCO problem. Better understanding of the PCO biomaterial effect added to the enhancing of the biomechanical effect will be the forefront of new lens technology in the future.

3. The biocompatibility of newer IOLs in general is excellent. However, there is a difference between materials. This is especially important for high risk patients such as those with a history of uveitis, or patients who have combined cataract and glaucoma surgery. At this point, it would appear that the hydrophilic acrylic group of IOLs followed closely by Allergan Phacoflex II SLM2 silicone, then heparin-surfaced modified PMMA, and AcrySof respectively, are all better than PMMA. It would appear first-generation silicone is worse than PMMA.

4. Concern about why people have unwanted images (dysphotopsia) post implantation and how to avoid these was first raised as a significant issue with oval IOLs with heightened concern about the mirror effect created by the flattened edge of AcrySof IOLs. All IOLs create dysphotopsia in some patients. The ability to mitigate

Figure 12-5a. Silicone IOL with silicone oil. (Figure courtesy of Hans Hoerauf, MD, Medizinische Universität zu Lubeck.)

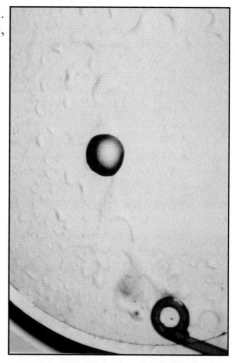

Figure 12-5b. Same IOL with silicone oil after rinsing with 044. (Figure courtesy of Hans Hoerauf, MD, Medizinische Universität zu Lubeck.)

dysphotopsia while adding desired features, such as a flattened edge for PCO prevention, will be an interesting exercise. However, we will never get better if we deny the problem and do not recognize this is an important patient outcome issue for at least a minority of our patients. I expect we will also see some progress here.

5. Wound size will approach a level where little is gained by incremental decreases in size. We found moving from a 4.0 mm to a 3.0 mm wound had a significant impact in regard to wound stability. We need to know more about this subject.

6. Other material concerns, such as the water vacuoles in AcrySof and the silicone oil problem with silicone lenses, are issues that need resolution. The chronic vacuoles in AcrySof are clearly different from the acute vacuoles associated with the Acrypak system. We need to know more about what is occurring with time, and the clinical significance of this problem. Fortunately, in regard to the silicone oil concern, it would appear that simple solvents used at the time of posterior segment surgery will resolve this issue. I expect technological advances to make both issues moot in the future.

The future is bright with our present results, which are expected to be even better. Due to the high level of patient satisfaction overall, expect relatively minor issues to move the market.

References

1. Neumann AC, Cobb B: Advantages and limitations of current soft intraocular lenses. J Cataract Refract Surg. 1989;15(3):257-263.

2. Bath PE, Boerner CF, Dang Y. Pathology and physics of YAG-laser intraocular lens damage. J Cataract Refract Surg. 1987;13:47-49.

3. Milauskas AT. Silicone intraocular lens implant discoloration in humans [letter]. Arch Ophthalmol. 109:913; reply 915, 1991.

4. Masket S, Garaghty E, Crandall AS, et al. Undesired light images associated with ovoid intraocular lenses. J Cataract Refract Surg. 1993;19:690-694.

5. Olson RJ, Crandall AS. Prospective randomized comparison of phacoemulsification cataract surgery with a 3.2 vs a 5.5 mm sutureless incision. Amer J Ophthalmol. 1998;125:612-620.

6. Leaming DV. Practice styles and preferences of ASCRS members—1998 survey. J Cataract Refract Surg. 1999;25:851-859.

7. Olson RJ, Crandall AS. Silicone versus polymethylmethacrylate intraocular lenses with regard to capsular opacification. Ophthalmol Surg Lasers. 1999;29(1):55-58.

8. Hayashi H, Hayashi K, Nakao F. Quantitative comparison of posterior capsule opacification after polymethylmethacrylate, silicone and soft acrylic intraocular lens implantation. Arch Ophthalmol. 1998;116:1579-1582.

9. Kumar R, Reeves DL, Olson RJ. Wound complications associated with incision enlargement when placing foldable intraocular lenses during cataract surgery. J Cataract Refract Surg. In press.

10. Hollick EJ, Spalton DJ, Ursell PG, et al. The effect of polymethylmethacrylate, silicone and polyacrylic intraocular lenses on posterior capsule opacification three years after cataract surgery. Ophthalmology. 1999;106:49-55.

11. Nishi O, Nishi K, Sakanishi K. Inhibition of migrating lens epithelial cells at the capsular bend created by the rectangular optic edge of a posterior chamber intraocular lens. Ophthalmic Surg Lasers. 1998;29:587-594.

12. Nishi O, Nishi K. Preventing posterior capsule opacification by creating a discontinuous sharp bend in the capsule. *J Cataract Refract Surg*. 1999;25(4):521-526.

13. Nishi O. The discontinuous capsular bend (sharp implant edge) rationale and experimental evidence. Paper presented at:The 1999 meeting of the European Society of Cataract and Refractive Surgeons; Vienna, Austria.

14. Hollick EJ, Spalton DJ, Ursell PG. Surface cytologic features on intraocular lenses: can increased biocompatibility have disadvantages? *Arch Ophthalmol*. 1999;117:872-878.

15. Versura P, Torreggiani A, Cellini M, et al. Adhesion mechanisms of human lens epithelial cells on 4 intraocular lens materials. *J Cataract Refract Surg*. 25:527-533.

16. Masket S. Cataract surgical problem, consultation section. *J Cataract Refract Surg*. 1997;23:979-984.

17. Farbowitz MA, Zabriskie NA, Crandall AS, et al. Visual complaints of patients with AcrySof acrylic intraocular lenses. *J Cataract Refract Surg*. In press.

18. Holladay JT, Lang A, Portney V. Analysis of edge glare phenomena in intraocular lens edge designs. *J Cataract and Refract Surg*. 1999;25(6);748-752.

20. Tester R, Olson RJ, Pace NL, et al. Dysphotopsia in phakic and pseudophakic patients—incidence and relation to commonly used intraocular lenses. *J Cataract Refract Surg*. In press.

21. Davison JA. What causes idiopathic temporal deposits? *Ocular Surgery News*. 1999;17:102-103.

22. Dhaliwal DK, Olson RJO, Mamalis N, et al. Visual significance of "glistenings" seen in the AcrySof lens. *J Cataract Refract Surg*. 1996;22:452-457.

23.. Omar OH, Pirayesh A, Mamalis N, et al. In vitro analysis of AcrySof intraocular lens "glistenings" in AcryPak and wagonwheel packaging. *J Cataract Refract Surg*. 1998;24:107-113.

24. Mitooka K, Hiroshi T, Takuya S. Glistening in acrylic IOLs. Paper presented at The ASCRS Symposium on Cataract, IOL, and Refractive Surgery; April 10-14, 1999; Seattle, Wash.

25. Christiansen G, Durcan FJ, Olson RJ, et al. Prevalence, severity, and visual significance of glistenings seen in the AcrySof intraocular lens one to four years from implantation. *J Cataract Refract Surg*. In press.

26. Hollick EJ, Spalton DJ, Ursell PG, et al. Biocompatibility of poly (methyl methacrylate), silicone, and AcrySof intraocular lenses: randomized comparison of the cellular reaction on the anterior lens surface. *J Cataract Refract Surg*. 1998;24:352-360.

27. Ravalico G, Baccara F, Lovisato A, et al. Postoperative cellular reaction on various intraocular lens materials. *Ophthalmology*. 1997;104:1084-1091.

28. Samuelson TW, Chu YR, Kreiger RA. Prospective randomized evaluation of giant cell deposits on foldable IOLs following combined cataract and glaucoma surgery. *J Cataract Refract Surgery*. In press.

29. Kumar R, Reeves DL, Brodstein D, Olson RJ. The MemoryLens: Protection of the retina during insertion. *J Cataract Refract Surg*. In Press.

30. Sugar J, Mitchelson J, Kraff M. Endothelial trauma and cell loss from intraocular lens insertion. *Arch Ophthalmol*. 1978;96(3):449-450.

31. Forstot SL, Blackwell WL, Jaffe NS, et al. The effect of intraocular lens implantation on the corneal endothelium. *Trans Am Acad Ophthalmol Otolaryngol*. 1977;83:195.

32. Kraff MC, Sanders DR, Lieberman HL, et al. Membrane formation after implantation of the polyvinyl alcohol-coated intraocular lenses. *Am Intraocular Imp Soc J*. 1980;6:129-136.

33. Borgioli M, Coster DJ, Ran RF, et al. Effect of heparin surface modification of polymethylmethacrylate intraocular lenses on signs of postoperative inflammation after extracapsular cataract extraction. One-year results of a double-masked multicenter study. *Ophthalmology*. 1992;99:1248-1254.

34. Lundgren B, Selen G, Spangberg M, et al. Fibrinous reaction on implanted intraocular lenses. A comparison of conventional PMMA and heparin surface modified lenses. *J Cataract Refract Surg.* 1992;18:236-239.

35. Memmen JE. The cataract wound, how big is it, really?! Paper presented at the Royal Hawaiian Eye Meeting; Hawaii, January 24-29, 1999.

36. Apple DJ, Isaacs RT, Kent DG, et al. Silicone oil adhesion to intraocular lenses: An experimental study comparing various biomaterials. *J Cataract Refract Surg.* 1997;23:536-544.

37. Hoerauf H, Menz D-H, Dresp J, et al. Use of 044 as a solvent for silicone oil adhesions on intraocular lenses. *J Cataract Refract Surg.* 1999;25:1292-1392.

38. Werner L, Escobar-Gomez M, Visessook N, et al. Histopathological study of anterior capsule opacification with different IOLs. Paper presented at The American Academy of Ophthalmology meeting. October 26, 1999; Orlando, Fla.

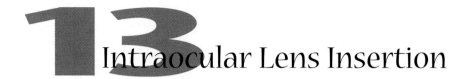

13 Intraocular Lens Insertion

Louis D. Nichamin, MD

As we embark upon the new millennium, the world of ophthalmology recently hailed a celebration of its own: the 50th anniversary of Sir Harold Ridley's original intraocular lens implant. More recently, a lesser but significant revolution has taken place in the US: the eclipsing of rigid IOL use by that of foldable lenses. Along with vast improvements in soft biomaterials and lens designs, there have also been marked advances in foldable IOL delivery systems.

Historically, pioneers in the field of foldable implants such as Epstein, Mazzocco, Levy, Faulkner, and others worked with bulky and unwieldy folding and inserting instruments or rudimentary injectors. Insertion of these lenses was inconsistent and at times frankly traumatic. The following discussion will review the latest refinements in IOL delivery devices.

SILICONE

Silicone, until recently, was considered the mainstay biomaterial used in foldable implants and continues to enjoy widespread use today. The choice of an optimal delivery system depends upon the particular elastomer employed, the material's refractive index (and hence its thickness), and perhaps most importantly, lens design.

Three-Piece Designs

Early silicone implants were comprised of a low index of refraction elastomers, and their central optic thickness was greater than that of more recent IOLs. Central optic thickness would vary depending upon dioptric power and could be quite thick for high power IOLs, making handling quite a challenging task. For this reason, manual inserting instrumentation had to be quite robust in design, and great care had to be directed toward proper loading and inserting.

Newer elastomers boast higher refractive indices and, therefore, maintain thinner profiles. This is enhanced across the dioptric range by allowing the effective optical zone to vary slightly based upon lens power; smaller zones are utilized for higher powers. These

Figure 13-1a. 6 to
12 o'clock fold.

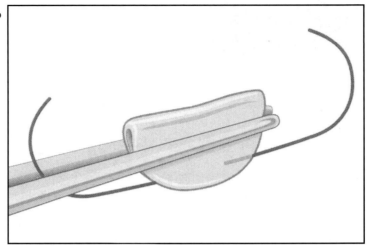

Figure 13-1b. 3 to
9 o'clock fold.

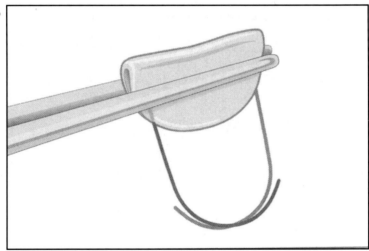

thinner lenses can be securely grasped and inserted with slimmer instruments, permitting placement through smaller incisions.

There are three basic orientations by which a three-piece IOL may be folded: 6 to 12, 3 to 9, or 4 to 10 o'clock (Figures 13-1a, 13-1b, and 13-1c). Certain implant designs (particularly haptic shape and its staking to the lens optic) favor one approach over another. Some surgeons prefer a 3 to 9, or 4 to 10 o'clock fold since both haptics will release simultaneously into the capsular bag. This technique is, however, potentially more traumatic, as haptic sweep could injure the posterior capsule. A 6 to 12 o'clock fold with manual placement of the trailing haptic is preferred in the setting of a compromised capsule or zonular apparatus.

When manually folding a silicone implant, care must be taken to keep both the implant and instrumentation dry since the surface of the silicone can be quite slippery. As with all implants, the optic should be placed flat on the loading platform, not tilted or teetering, and well-centered within the loading device (Figure 13-2). If an uneven fold occurs, the loading should be repeated.

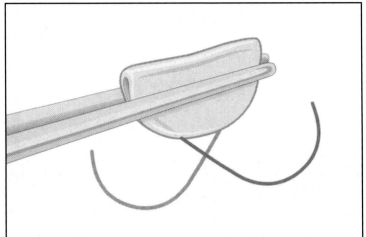

Figure 13-1c. 4 to 10 o'clock.

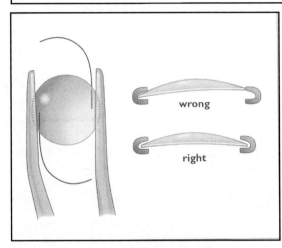

Figure 13-2. Proper folding of three-piece loop haptic IOLs requires that the implant be flat on the loading surface and well-centered within the loading device.

wrong

right

Historically, injector delivery systems for three-piece IOLs were fraught with problems, often leading to unpredictable if not traumatic delivery of implants. Recently, however, a new generation of delivery devices has emerged that have been engineered to allow for remarkably safe, facile, and reproducible placement of these implants. The first of these devices to reach the marketplace was the Unfolder, produced by Allergan Medical Optics. The Silver series is used to deliver the SI 30, SI 40, and SA 40N Array multifocal implants (all 6.0 mm optics) through potentially unenlarged phaco incisions (Figure 13-3a). The Gold series handpiece and cartridge are similar and used for the 5.5 mm SI 55 IOL and may be placed through even smaller incisions (Figure 13-3b). These metal-threaded-injectors incorporate a soft silicone-tipped plunger that advances the optic and allows for placement of the trailing haptic (Figure 13-3c). The metal threads have recently been enlarged, increasing the speed of delivery of the IOL. These injectors require partial rotation along their long axes during delivery for consistent and properly oriented implant placement.

The Mport, manufactured by Bausch & Lomb Surgical, is used to deliver their model LI61-U three-piece silicone implant. It consists of a plastic disposable syringe-style device

Figure 13-3a. The AMO Silver Unfolder used to deliver the 6.0 mm silicone mon and multifocal implants.

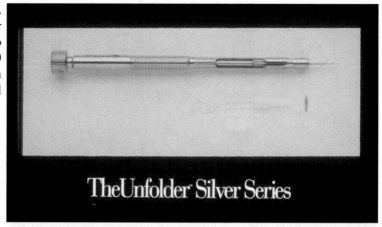

Figure 13-3b. The AMO Gold Unfolder used to deliver the 5.5 mm SI 55 IOL.

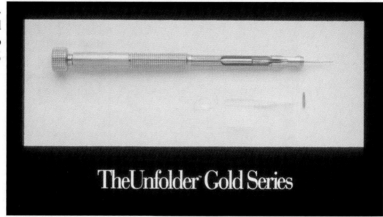

Figure 13-3c. The soft silicone-tipped plunger advances the lens optic and can deliver the trailing haptic.

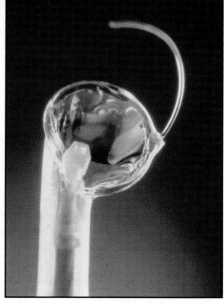

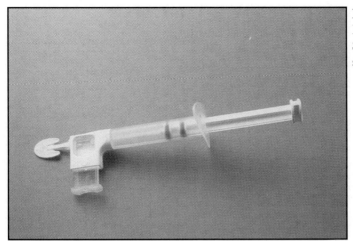

Figure   13-4a. The Bausch   &   Lomb Surgical Mport syringe-style injector.

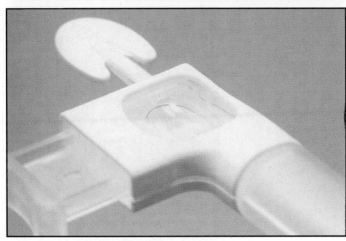

Figure 13-4b. Closure of the loading drawer compresses the optic into an "M" configuration.

that allows for one-handed delivery without rotation of the device. It has the unique quality of compressing the lens optic into an "M" configuration (Figures 13-4a, 13-4b, and 13-4c). Following placement of the lens optic, its plunger may also be retracted and used to insert the trailing haptic. It is currently undergoing downsizing to allow for placement through incision sizes of 3.0 mm or less.

Plate Haptic Designs

Single-piece plate haptic silicone implants have lost some of their popularity recently due to improvements in three-piece designs and newer biomaterials. They have, however, enjoyed much success over the years in large part due to their ease of insertion and small associated incision sizes. The only approved toric IOL in the United States is the Staar Surgical silicone plate design; therefore, this general lens design continues to occupy an important position among our current armamentarium. Both threaded and syringe-style injectors exist for this lens style and allow for placement through incision sizes of 2.8 mm or less (Figure 13-5).

Figure   13-4c.
Depression of the
plunger affords delivery of the implant in a
flat, planar orientation.

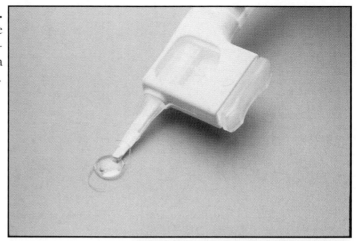

Figure 13-5. Staar Surgical syringe and threaded injectors used to implant their single-piece plate haptic IOLs.

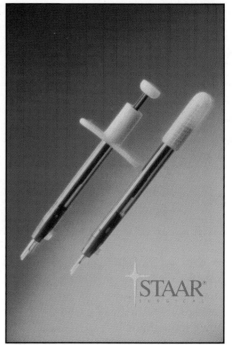

ACRYLIC

Soft acrylic has become a very popular biomaterial today and is utilized in the Alcon AcrySof and Allergan Sensar IOLs. Because of the AcrySof's thermoelastic properties, mild warming of the lens is commonly employed to soften the implant and facilitate folding and release. This material, unlike silicone, may be wetted with BSS or viscoelastic and will aid in handling, since the surface of this implant is tacky and prone to surface marring. Inserting instrumentation should be smooth and free of burrs or scratches. The implant may be folded by using the disposable Acrypak produced by Alcon (Figures 13-6a and 13-6b) or by conventional instrumentation. By pressing centrally on the under-

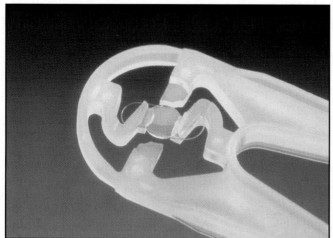

Figure 13-6a. The Alcon disposable AcryPak loader.

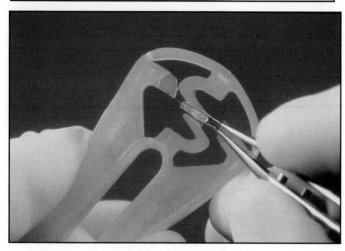

Figure 13-6b. After squeezing the loader, the implant is grasped with inserting forceps.

surface of the optic as the fold is initiated, a proper inverted "U" configuration is achieved. Inserting forceps designed by Buratto or Lehner are popular since they minimize contact with the delicate central optic surface. As compared to a folded silicone lens, the acrylic optic should be grasped a little lower, toward the open aspect of the fold, to avoid "fish-mouthing" of the optic edges. The 5.5 mm AcrySof optic generally requires a 3.2 mm incision, and the 6.0 mm optic will pass through a 3.8 mm incision.

Recently, Alcon has released the Monarch injector delivery system for both their MA 30 5.5 mm three-piece design lens as well as their newly introduced SA 30 one-piece design. It permits excellent visualization of the folding process and implant delivery. It is a metal-threaded device and requires a 3.5 to 3.8 mm incision (Figure 13-7).

The recently approved Allergan Sensar acrylic IOL is delivered through their Sapphire injector, specifically designed for this implant (Figures 13-8a and 13-8b). It requires an approximate 3.2 mm incision.

Figure 13-7. The Alcon Monarch delivery system.

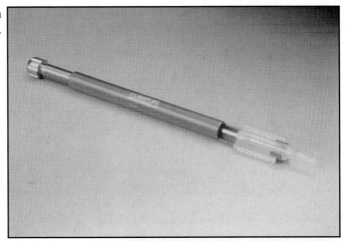

Figure 13-8a. The AMO Sensar acrylic implant.

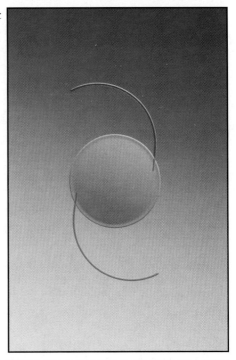

Figure 13-8b. The Sapphire Injector delivery system.

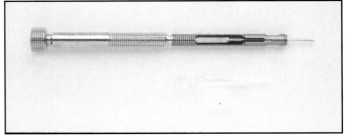

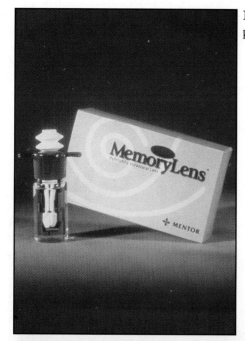

Figure 13-9a. The Mentor Memory Lens packaged in a prerolled configuration.

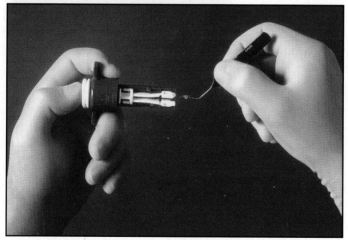

Figure 13-9b. Removal of the lens.

HYDROGEL

This category of hydrophilic acrylic implants currently has two FDA approved lenses. The first, the Mentor Memory Lens, is the only IOL that is available pre-rolled from the manufacturer, obviating the need to fold the implant (Figures 13-9a, 13-9b, and 13-9c). It is simply removed from its package and inserted directly into the incision. Kelman-McPherson or similar forceps will suffice for insertion, or specifically designed instruments may be used to help minimize incision size and improve holding power upon the grasped optic. Typical incision sizes are 3.8 mm. As the leading haptic is being placed, care must be taken to angle in a clockwise direction so that the broad C-shaped haptics

Figure 13-9c. Grasped with forceps, the implant may be inserted with no other folding or loading maneuvers.

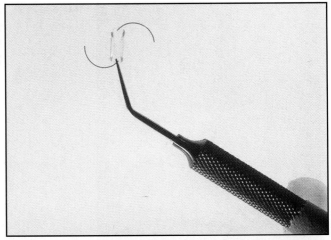

Figure 13-10a. The Bausch & Lomb Surgical Hydroview IOL.

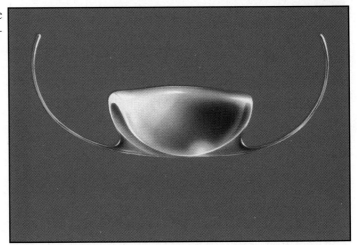

are properly positioned under the anterior capsular leaflet. The trailing haptic is placed in a conventional manner. Unfolding of the optic then takes place over several minutes. One need not wait to visualize the lens' final position.

The other recently approved implant in this family is the Bausch & Lomb Hydroview. This IOL, by virtue of its bonded haptics, is said to behave more as a one-piece design. It is currently being marketed internationally in conjunction with the Surefold delivery system (Figures 13-10a and 13-10b). After squeezing the disposable Surefold, the lens is folded along its 6 to 12 o'clock axis. It is then grasped and inserted with simple forceps. Folding in any other orientation risks damage to the bonded haptics. Incision size will range from 3.5 to 3.8 mm depending upon IOL power.

AVOIDING TROUBLE

Most complications that occur when inserting a foldable implant are related to one of two problems: either the implant was not loaded properly into the folding/loading device or the surgeon attempted to force the IOL through too small of an incision.

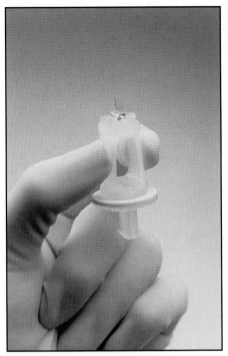

Figure 13-10b. The Surefold loader, provided in the disposable packaging, folds the implant in the proper 6 to 12 o'clock orientation.

The first problem can, of course, be avoided by devoting the necessary attention to the details of the loading process. As previously mentioned, when manually folding and loading a three-piece implant, care must be taken to ensure that the lens is flat on the loading surface. If it is tilted, then an uneven fold will likely occur, which then may result in premature release from the inserting forceps. Most loading devices have demarcations or "hash marks" to help align the center of the lens optic with the center of the loading device. Similar care must be given to the centering and positioning of an implant when using an injector delivery device.

When it comes to incision size, most surgeons would agree that smaller is better. Unfortunately, forcing an implant through an inadequately enlarged incision has been shown to traumatize the wound and potentially compromise its ability to self-seal. In addition, one risks premature release of the implant with subsequent ocular injury and/or damage to the implant.

CONCLUSION

Today's phaco surgeon now has a number of choices with regard to foldable intraocular lenses. One's ultimate choice will depend upon the optical performance of the lens, its biocompatibility, its associated incision size, and not least of which is its ease of insertion. Fortunately, the latest generation of delivery devices has greatly improved the facility and reproducibility of inserting contemporary small incision implants.

14 Reducing Astigmatism

Louis D. Nichamin, MD
R. Bruce Wallace III, MD

To become less dependent on glasses after implanting an intraocular lens, especially a multifocal lens, astigmatism must be reduced.[1] Fortunately, the surgical correction of corneal astigmatism has been improving and has been rapidly gaining in popularity. Today, many patients become relatively free of astigmatism thanks to these new remedies.

ASTIGMATISM IN THREE DIMENSIONS

In order to reduce unwanted astigmatism, surgeons must lead the way in their practice to develop a systematic approach to surgical correction. Reducing astigmatism begins with effective preoperative assessment. Most cataract surgeons depend on trained technicians to perform preoperative astigmatism measurements, which include refraction, keratometry, and videokeratography or corneal topography. Unfortunately, most technicians do not think about astigmatism in three dimensions because these measurements only generate numbers or two-dimensional color maps. However, for technicians and surgeons to be effective in astigmatism control, it is helpful to understand and visualize astigmatism, especially corneal astigmatism, in three dimensions. Such terms as the "flat axis," the "steep axis," and "coupling" become easier to grasp when thinking of corneal shapes rather than numbers or colors.

To determine if your office staff perceives astigmatism in three dimensions, try this experiment. Ask your best-trained technicians to imagine that the oblong curvatures of an American football represent the astigmatic corneal surfaces of a patient's eye with the curvature in one axis steep, the other flat. Imagine that the football is lying flat on the ground. Would that resemble with-the-rule or against-the-rule astigmatism? If they answer with-the-rule, they are correct and are probably thinking about astigmatism in three dimensions (unless they are just good guessers). With this fundamental understanding of what the term "regular astigmatism" means, all members of the surgical team will find astigmatism correction easier to understand.

INCISION DECISIONS

Over the past several years, a great deal of effort has centered upon the study of the astigmatic effects of various cataract incisions. By manipulating incision parameters (size, location, and shape) surgeons could, with a reasonable level of accuracy, "tailor" their astigmatic outcome according to the patient's preexisting astigmatism. This on-axis, variable incisional approach does however require effort rotating about the operating room table, a dynamic mindset and, to some degree, varying instrumentation. Although effective, recent advances in incisional technique and implant technology have led to a different approach in managing astigmatism during phaco surgery. Specifically, the temporal clear corneal phaco incision, as popularized by Dr. Howard Fine, has now been proven to be safe, effective, and remarkably reproducible. Additionally, as a result of improvements in foldable IOL delivery systems, implantation may now be routinely performed through incisions of 3.0 to 3.2 mm.

Well-documented studies now support the clinical impression that incisions of this size behave in an essentially astigmatically neutral fashion.[2,3] Thus, an incision that yields all of the wonderful benefits of the clear corneal approach, yet is astigmatically neutral, may now be easily and reproducibly crafted. If a patient has enough preexisting astigmatism to warrant reduction, modern astigmatic keratotomy may then be conservatively added to arrive at the desired cylindrical outcome.

Admittedly, this approach may result in a greater number of incisions placed onto the cornea. However, use of peripheral (intralimbal), arcuate, astigmatic, relaxing incisions has proven to be extremely safe and reliable. In the setting of concomitant cataract surgery, our data indicate that this technique provides for more predictable astigmatic outcomes as compared to the use of conventional (smaller) AK optical zones and yields more consistent results than when relying solely upon a "tailored" phaco incision.

Our use of limbal arcuate relaxing incisions originated from the work of Dr. Stephen Hollis. With refinement of his nomogram, we found this approach to astigmatic keratotomy to be considerably more forgiving with less induced shift of resultant cylinder axis and greater predictability. This heightened safety level makes the technique most appropriate for the cataract-aged population in which overcorrection should generally be avoided. Furthermore, this form of intralimbal keratotomy seems to logically dovetail with the trend toward clear corneal phaco incisions. Thus, we start with the amazingly simple but elegant single-plane, beveled (neutral) clear corneal phaco incision, and then add to it the necessary nonbeveled (perpendicular to the corneal surface) limbal arcuate relaxing incisions. This makes for a facile, logical, and aesthetic approach to astigmatism management.

SURGICAL PLANNING

The goal for astigmatism control should be the creation of a resultant cylinder of less than 1 D at any axis. Most patients enjoy good unaided visual acuity with this degree of astigmatism. Some studies suggest a benefit to leaving some amount of residual against-the-rule cylinder so that uncorrected near vision after cataract surgery is improved.[4,5] However, surgical practices utilizing multifocal IOLs and/or monovision will not find this to be an advantage because of the compromise of the loss of distance visual acuity with amounts over 1 D of cylinder.

One of the more challenging tasks that the surgeon faces is deciding which astigmatic preoperative measurements should be used when planning a surgical correction. Do we depend on the cylinder diopters and axis from the refraction, the keratometry, or do we always need to perform corneal topography? One study showed the frequency of poor correlation of all three methods of measurement, especially with less than 2 D of astigmatism.[6] Fortunately, unlike correction of spherical refractive errors, astigmatism correction is more forgiving, especially when treating moderate to low levels.

One way to plan surgical correction of astigmatism is to initially assess the refraction and the keratometry simultaneously. If good correlation exists as to the amount of cylinder and axis, planning astigmatism correction during cataract surgery is fairly straightforward. If, however, there is poor correlation (even though keratometry should be more reliable), surgical correction can be less predictable, even with corneal topography. This is where the "art" of astigmatism correction applies. The surgeon needs to also judge the relative reliability of the astigmatic information. If after careful consideration there is doubt as to a reasonable surgical plan, the astigmatism correction should be postponed until after cataract surgery and an adequate time for wound healing.

Phaco surgery is performed through a 2.5 mm to 3.0 mm incision, depending upon the tip and sleeve combination, and then may need to be enlarged to 3.2 mm to 3.4 mm to accommodate a particular foldable IOL. This single plane, paracentesis-style, temporal incision is placed at or just anterior to the vascular arcade. If a larger incision is to be used (to accommodate a particular IOL), increased against-the-wound drift (with-the-rule astigmatism, given temporal incision location) must be anticipated and factored into the amount of cylinder to be corrected. As seen in the following nomograms, for patients with minimal preexisting astigmatism the single plane phaco incision is employed. For patients with mild against-the-rule astigmatism, a nasal peripheral, arcuate, relaxing incision is placed opposite to the temporal clear corneal phaco incision leading to a neat, symmetrical corneal flattening. For moderate levels, a temporal arcuate incision is placed along with the nasal incision. This temporal cut, in essence, becomes a deep groove such that the incision architecture resembles the Langerman hinge (with the extent or length of the groove determined by the nomogram).

For with-the-rule astigmatism, the surgeon has two choices. There is varying opinion regarding the safety of superior clear corneal incisions. Many leading surgeons fully advocate their use. It is generally acceptable to use a superior clear corneal incision provided that the patient has at least 2 D of with-the-rule cylinder and good globe exposure. This most commonly occurs in young, myopic patients. One must keep in mind that these superior incisions will drift against the wound more than temporal incisions, as noted by Dr. Harry Grabow, et al.[7] In most cases of with-the-rule astigmatism, it is best to keep the phaco tunnel situated temporally, maintain an incision size of 3.5 mm or less for neutrality, and apply astigmatic keratotomy incisions over the steep axis. In our experience, this approach has yielded more consistent results with less corneal edema, particularly in those patients who have short eyes with small corneal diameters, are deeply set, or have compromised endothelium. A final planning note for patients who have with-the-rule astigmatism: the side-port incision location may need to be adjusted so as not to interfere with the intralimbal relaxing incision.

Figure 14-1. Performing a limbal relaxing incision with a single foot plate diamond knife.

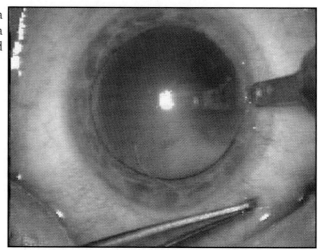

SURGICAL TECHNIQUE

The actual technique begins with verification of the steep meridian using intraoperative keratoscopy. Formerly, we would place all AK incisions at the conclusion of surgery, in the event that a complication necessitated a modification to the phaco incision. For routine cases, we now prefer to place these incisions at the outset in order to avoid epithelial disruption. One exception would be in the case of high against-the-rule astigmatism where the nomogram calls for a long temporal arcuate incision. If this incision or "groove" is placed to its full arc length prior to phacoemulsification, significant gaping and edema may result secondary to intraoperative manipulation. In this situation, the temporal incision is made by first creating a two-plane, grooved phaco incision (600 micron depth), which is then extended to the full arc length, as determined by the nomogram at the conclusion of surgery. The nasal arc may be extended to its full arc length at the beginning of the case.

The astigmatic incisions are placed just inside of the limbus at an empiric depth of 600 microns (Figure 14-1). Prior studies employing pachymetry and adjusted blade settings yielded negligible benefit in this older population, as opposed to younger refractive surgery patients where variable blade depth settings may be justified. Diamond blade style and configuration may require an adjustment in depth settings. For one of us (Nichamin), a triple-edged 15 degree Thornton arcuate diamond set at this depth has yielded excellent results with no perforations. A new diamond blade solely dedicated to this technique is now available from Mastel. A single footplate improves visibility and the diamond extends to the appropriate (600 micron) preset depth. The similarly designed single footplate trifacet diamond knife made by Mastel, the "John Groover," has also been effective. Similar designs are available from Rhein Medical and Storz.

The extent of arc to be incised may be demarcated in several different ways. One method makes use of a specially designed Fine-Thornton fixation ring that both fixates the globe and allows one to delineate the extent of arc by visually extrapolating from the limbus to the adjacent marker (Mastel Precision and Rhein Medical, Tampa, Fla). Each incremental mark is 10 degrees apart, and bold marks 180 degrees apart serve to align with the steep axis. This approach avoids inking and marking of the cornea. If desired, a

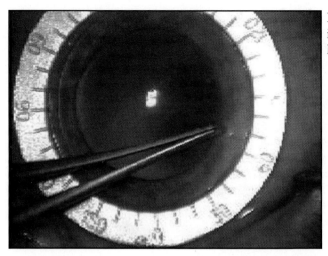

Figure 14-2. Marking the intended incision site for a limbal relaxing incision.

two-cut RK marker may be lightly inked and used to mark the exact extent of arc to be incised in conjunction with the fixation ring/gauge (See Figure 14-2). Alternatively, a Thornton-Nichamin arcuate marker utilizing a 10 mm optical zone may be used to mark the cornea (Moria, imported by Microtech, Doylestown, Pa).

Increased Comfort for Patient and Doctor

Interestingly, one of the most common patient complaints following contemporary phaco surgery is that of a foreign body sensation. Intralimbal relaxing incisions, as compared to more central corneal incisions (smaller optical zones), definitely improve patient comfort. With the addition of a postoperative topical NSAID, this problem is virtually eliminated. Upon examination, these incisions appear to heal quickly and are nearly unidentifiable within several days.

Conclusion

This approach to astigmatism management has been evolving for the past 5 years and parallels the development of several similar techniques, such as Dr. Robert Kershner's keratolenticuloplasty technique and Dr. Jim Gills' use of LRIs. Through these techniques, both patient and surgeon may enjoy the great benefit of clear corneal surgery performed through an unenlarged phaco incision in concert with a safe and reproducible means to correct preexisting astigmatism.

Once again, acknowledgement is given to Dr. Stephen Hollis of Columbus, Ga, whose original work provided the platform for this technique, and to Dr. Spencer Thornton, who has contributed so much to astigmatism surgery and whose modifiers are incorporated into this current nomogram. Drs. David Dillman and William Maloney have also shared in the evolution of these astigmatic procedures.

REFERENCES

1. Knorz M, Koch D, Marinez-Franco C, Lorger C. Effect of pupil size and astigmatism on contrast acuity with monofocal and bifocal intraocular lenses. *J Cataract Refract Surg.* 1994; 20:26-33.

2. Lyle W, Jin G. Prospective evaluation of early visual and refractive effects with small clear corneal incision for cataract surgery. *J Cataract Refract Surg.* 1996;22:1456-1460.

3. Masket S, Tennen D. Astigmatic stabilization of 3.0 mm temporal clear corneal cataract incisions. *J Cataract Refract Surg.* 1996;22:1451-1455.

4. Verzella F, Calossi A. Multifocal effect of against-the-rule myopic astigmatism in pseudophakic eyes. *J Refract Corneal Surg.* 1993;9:58-61.

5. Sawusch M, Guyton D. Optimal astigmatism to enhance depth of focus after cataract surgery. *Ophthalmology.* 1991;98:1025-1029.

6. Wallace RB. On–axis cataract incisions: where is the axis? *1995 ASCRS Symposium of Cataract, IOL and Refractive Surgery Best Papers of Sessions.* Nov. 1995; 67-72.

15 Creating Multifocality

R. Bruce Wallace III, MD

The inevitable loss of near vision in the aging human population is usually not painful, dangerous, or tragic. The gradual onset of presbyopia allows its victims more time to adjust to this unwanted curse, accept the limitations it creates, and the unpopular adjustments it requires. Wearing bifocal glasses or half-reading glasses is now considered the natural result of getting older.

Bifocal glasses, an over 200-year-old technology, always cause loss of distance vision with inferior gaze and do not allow for improved near vision except with inferior gaze. Added to these optical limitations are the nuisance and cosmetic compromise of spectacle dependency. How often have patients shown any happiness toward "needing bifocals"? Bifocals are becoming even less popular during this age of refractive surgery. With new developments in laser vision correction, patients are lining up to rid their need for glasses. Yet, for many, this will only mean less need for glasses for distance vision. The pre-presbyope patient undergoing refractive surgery to improve uncorrected distance vision generally ignores the fact that his or her loss of near vision in the years ahead will require him or her to return to glasses. With the rapid expansion of electronic communication and the increase in time spent at the computer (not to mention longer life spans), good near vision will be essential. Consequently, methods to improve uncorrected near vision will be receiving a lot more attention.

Since presbyopia is so common, why haven't we been able to find a universal remedy? Well, for one thing, we are not certain as to how accommodation really works. Many theories exist going back to Helmholtz.[1] A recent theory is that the crystalline lens just keeps getting bigger as we get older and the zonules lose their taughtness and therefore are less effective in changing the shape of the lens. Schachar has advocated radial incisions in the anterior equatorial sclera to expand the ciliary body and restore zonular tension.[2] While this may help the early presbyope, some wonder what effect, if any, nuclear sclerosis will have on limiting accommodation even after this type of procedure. Other methods have been (and continue to be) considered to restore multifocality. Simple corneal astigmatism, which can be created surgically, can increase depth of field and marginally improve near vision, though at the compromise of reduced uncorrected distance vision.[3-5] Various spring action and hinged IOLs have been investigated to restore near vision after crystalline lens removal.[6-8]

Aside from various bifocal contact lenses, monovision has been the most widely accepted method used to restore multifocality. Despite its popularity, very little is understood as to just how to maximize monovision. Most eye care providers correct the dominant eye for distance and the nondominant eye for near, but not all patients prefer this arrangement. A certain percentage of monovision trials are unsuccessful. Predicting success is not easy, even with contact lens trials. Pre-presbyopes have an especially difficult time adjusting to monovision after refractive surgery, even though the long-term benefits are significant. Success with monovision depends on visual cortical adaptation, the suppression of unneeded and out-of-focus vision in the opposite eye of the eye in focus. In my experience, and in many others, monovision has been an incredibly useful tool to restore multifocality, though in a relatively unphysiologic way.[9]

Many cataract and refractive surgeons find the concept of monovision too time consuming to explain to preoperative candidates and patient acceptance too unpredictable. Potential loss of stereopsis has been another concern. In addition, some postoperative patients remain uncertain about their surgical result in the near eye when covering the distance eye while looking at distance objects. The hassle with the occasional unhappy patient has steered many cataract and refractive surgeons away from monovision.

Multifocal IOLs have now emerged as the first real competitor to monovision for the cataract patient interested in better near vision. Like monovision, multifocal IOLs can provide near acuity in all fields of gaze, not just inferior gaze as with bifocal glasses. This is a real advantage when trying to read information on an object positioned above eye level. Like monovision, multifocal IOLs require some degree of visual cortex adaptation. The patient's complex "plastic" brain cells need to adjust to a new visual system, suppress the unwanted out-of-focus image, and learn to ignore rings and halos.

Some important questions concerning multifocal IOL performance remain for many surgeons and their patients. Who are the best candidates? What information do patients need to know in order to make an informed decision before implantation? What steps can surgeons take to maximize patient satisfaction? The following chapters will hopefully help to broaden our understanding of multifocal IOLs and promote the benefits of refractive cataract surgery.

REFERENCES

1. Weale R. Presbyopia toward the end of the 20th century. *Surv Ophthalmol.* 1989;34:15-30.
2. Schachar R. Is Helmholtz's theory of accomodation correct? *Ann Ophthalmology.* 1999;31(1):10-17.
3. Wallace RB. *Multifocal Vision After Cataract Surgery.* Philadelphia, Pa: Rapid Science Publishers; 1998.
4. Verzella F, Calossi A. Multifocal effect of against-the-rule myopic astigmatism in pseudophakic eyes. *Refract Corneal Surg.* 1993;9:58-61.
5. Sawusch M, Guyton D. Optimal astigmatism to enhance depth of focus after cataract surgery. *Ophthalmology.* 1991;96:1025-1029.
6. Cumming JS, Kammann J. Experience with an accommodating IOL. *J Cataract Refract Surg.* 1996;22:1001.

7.   Hara T, Hara T, Yasuda A, Yamada Y. Accommodative intraocular lens with spring action. Part 1. Design and placement in an excised animal eye. *Ophthalmic Surgery.* 1990;21:128-133.

8.   Hara T, Hara T, Mizumoto Y. Accommodative intraocular lens with spring action. Part 2. Fixation in the living rabbit. *Ophthalmic Surgery.* 1992;23:632-635.

9.   Boerner C, Thrasher B. Results of monovision correction in bilateral pseudophakes. *Am Intra-Ocular Implant Soc J.* 1984;10:49-50.

16
Multifocal IOLs: Past and Present

R. Bruce Wallace III, MD

Present day attitudes toward multifocal IOL use remain mixed. However, a look back at the history of monofocal IOLs may help to better understand current opinion regarding multifocal IOLs.

Monofocal IOLs have enjoyed immense popularity over the past 20 years. Today, it is hard to justify not implanting an IOL during cataract surgery. Since aphakia has always been an unpopular and undesirable end result of cataract surgery, one would naturally jump to the conclusion that IOL implantation would spread like wildfire. Considering this fact, it's amazing how long it took for monofocal lens implants to gain general acceptance since the first IOL was implanted over 50 years ago.

For the first 30 years, most ophthalmologists viewed the IOL as risky, uncertain, and even unnecessary. The status quo of surgical aphakia was so familiar that many surgeons were reluctant to break with tradition and begin using IOLs. It is hard to believe that during the 1970s, many ophthalmologists expected extended wear soft contact lenses to overtake IOLs as the safest and most effective remedy for aphakia.

What happened to reverse this stubborn reluctance to endorse IOL implantation? Was it due to technological breakthroughs, better surgical techniques, and better IOL designs? Yes and no. Cataract surgery was enjoying a relative renaissance prior to IOL use. Thanks to Dr. Charles Kelman, phacoemulsification helped to shift surgeons from intracapsular cataract extraction (ICCE) to extracapsular cataract extraction (ECCE). By the mid 1970s, ECCE began to overtake ICCE as the method of choice for most cataract procedures worldwide. Few cataract surgeons were willing to perform phacoemulsification at first, opting for removal of the intact nucleus followed either manually by cortical removal or mechanically by taking advantage of the controlled irrigation and aspiration systems made available from phacoemulsification equipment manufacturers. With ECCE and phaco, the stage was set for iris plane capsular fixated IOL implantation, and finally, posterior chamber IOLs.

Certainly ECCE, phaco, and IOL design improvements helped to enhance the safety and predictability of IOL implantation. Yet, even after the ECCE technique was squarely positioned as the standard for cataract extraction and dependable posterior chamber IOLs (such as those designed by Drs. Sinsky, Kratz, Sheets, and Simcoe) were widely available, IOL implantation remained spotty.

However, as cataract surgeons began to witness the substantial patient satisfaction of pseudophakia over aphakia, the tide eventually shifted in favor of the IOL. At first, there were only rigid PMMA IOL styles available. Foldable silicone IOLs, introduced in the mid 1980s, took many years to become popular. In fact, each logical step in IOL improvement has faced a measure of skepticism and resistance to acceptance, similar to the attitudes many surgeons demonstrated during the early days of IOL development. One major catalyst kept IOL development moving forward: surgical aphakia needed a safe and effective cure.

As this evolutionary pattern of implant surgery continues to unfold, multifocal IOLs present surgeons with a new and important option for the visual rehabilitation of the cataract patient. A number of issues surrounding MIOL use have been cause for concern, principally the side effects of unwanted halos and the loss of contrast sensitivity. However, not all of the reluctance toward MIOL acceptance has been due to a fear of "doing harm" by creating unwanted visual sensations and decreased contrast sensitivity. For MIOLs to continue to grow in popularity, for designs to evolve, and for MIOLs to eventually dominate over monofocal IOLs, poor uncorrected near vision after cataract surgery will need to be considered an unacceptable result, similar to surgical aphakia. Refractive cataract surgery must begin to involve not only better uncorrected vision at distance but also intermediate and especially near vision before multifocal IOLs triumph over monofocal IOLs.

MULTIFOCAL IOL DEVELOPMENT

The pioneers of multifocal IOLs have included not only cataract surgeons but also a multitude of research scientists, optical physicists, engineers, study coordinators, statisticians, and clinical analysts. Years of dedication to research into optical designs and visual performance have been sacrificed in order to provide the best implant to effectively and safely restore multifocality.

Center Surround MIOL

In the US, the first MIOL product to be granted FDA investigational status (investigational device exemption or IDE) was the "center surround" or "bull's eye" lens manufactured by Precision-Cosmet and later acquired by the IOLAB Corporation. This PMMA MIOL had a central near add surrounded by a distance optical power. Empirically, the idea of implanting an MIOL with a near component in the center of the visual axis would seem likely to cause a significant and sudden loss of distance vision upon pupillary miosis. However, an early study reported by Keates and Pearce found that after measuring visual changes with the Brightness Acuity Tester (BAT) (Mentor Ophthalmics, Santa Barbara, Calif), distance visual acuities were adversely affected in only a small minority of eyes implanted with the Precision Cosmet/IOLAB MIOL.[1] The explanation for uninterrupted distance vision may be due to limited miosis or slight IOL decentration. Regardless of these clinical findings, most surgeons have considered this style of MIOL to be "near dominant".

As with all MIOLs, the center surround style did decrease contrast sensitivity when compared to monofocal IOLs. In a study by Ravalico, et al, noticeable loss of contrast sensitivity was found in eyes with this style MIOL compared to monofocal IOL eyes and phakic eyes.[2] Chiron, and later Bausch & Lomb, purchased this technology, now under

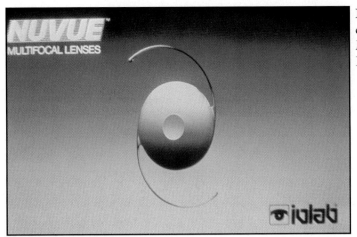

Figure 16-1. Nu-Vue center surround PMMA MIOL (Bausch & Lomb).

the name NuVue (Bausch & Lomb Surgical) (Figure 16-1). A foldable silicone NuVue has been designed, but further clinical investigation is pending.

Diffractive MIOL

The investigation of the center surround refractive MIOL was soon followed by the introduction of the diffractive MIOL by the 3M Corporation (St. Paul, Minn), with Dr. Richard Lindstrom appointed as medical monitor for US (FDA) studies. The first 3M diffractive MIOL was added to the Sheets posterior chamber IOL because of its excellent centration characteristics (the Sheets monofocal IOL was also one of the first posterior chamber IOLs to be devoid of fixation holes in the peripheral optic and to be designed for capsular bag fixation) (Figure 16-2).

Diffractive optics remain relatively unfamiliar to most cataract surgeons. Diffraction has actually been considered an optical flaw. Diffraction has two effects: destructive interference and constructive interference, and the theory of diffraction is centuries old. The wave theory of light was developed by Christiaan Huygens in the second half of the 17th century. From this theory, diffraction was discovered as a "double refraction," later explained by Young as constructive and destructive interference. The 3M diffractive IOL utilized the physical principles of diffraction and light wave "constructive interference" in conjunction with refraction to create two optical powers. The diffractive portion utilized discrete zone steps on the lens surface to control the wave property of light. The resultant waves created phase relationships so that a diffractive constructive interference produced a separate focal plane. The design consisted of a meniscus-shaped, 6 mm overall diameter optic with a smooth refractive anterior surface and a series of diffractive microstructure rings superimposed on the posterior surface. A major advantage of this approach was that the two dioptric powers were largely unaffected by pupil size and lens decentration.

The diffractive optic of this MIOL directed transmitted light to two primary focal points. Forty percent of light was devoted to distance vision, 40% to near, and 20% of light transmission was lost to higher orders of refraction. Incoming light could be incident on any portion of the two zones within the pupil and still produce two points of focus. For this reason, the diffractive lens could tolerate moderate amounts of decentration and

Figure 16-2. 3M diffractive PMMA MIOL (Alcon).

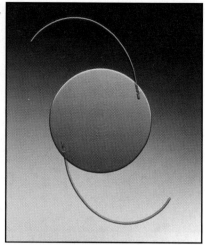

variation in pupil size.[3] All zones of the lens surface contributed to the dual power function, unlike a Fresnel lens of distinct refractive regions. In fact, according to Simpson, there may be distinct differences between a Fresnel prism, which is a refractive optic, and the diffractive plate of the 3M-Alcon MIOL.[4]

Lindstrom reported near vision results at 1-year postoperative implantation of the diffractive MIOL compared to monofocal IOLs. With distance correction only, eyes achieving J_1 to J_3 near acuity were found in 92% with MIOL, compared to 37% with monofocal IOL, and 59% of bilaterally implanted 3M diffractive MIOL patients never needed spectacles. There were no statistically significant differences in corrected distance or near visual acuity when compared to eyes with pupil sizes ranging from 2.0 mm to 7.0 mm.[5] Gimbel reported on 149 patients with bilateral 3M diffractive multifocal IOLs, finding 63% of patients needed no spectacle correction compared to 4% of monofocal cases. Multifocal patients reported significantly more visual side effects, such as glare and halos, and a greater decrease in contrast sensitivity at low contrast levels was detected among multifocal cases.[6] A German study demonstrated surprisingly high loss of contrast sensitivity for both 3M diffractive multifocal patients and monofocal patients. Seventy percent of MIOL patients and 56% of monofocal patients failed to meet the minimum requirements for a driver's license in Germany.[7]

Restoration of near vision with this multifocal IOL began to be called "pseudoaccommodation" and, as expected, patient satisfaction was highest when the distance refraction was near emmetropia and astigmatism was minimal. Low hyperopic patients were found to have fewer problems than low myopes.[8]

An FDA advisory panel recommended approval of the diffractive MIOL in 1992 if certain strict clinical evaluations of this lens were found satisfactory, such as visual performance under various driving conditions. This MIOL was purchased by Alcon Laboratories and named the RëStor lens. Recently, Alcon has been redesigning the diffractive optic to reduce the possibility of unwanted visual imagery and is considering adding this diffractive component to the popular AcrySof acrylic IOL. Other companies, such as

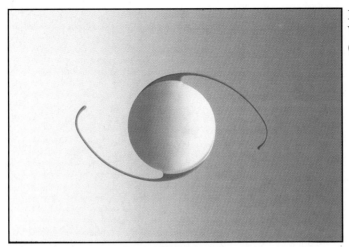

Figure 16-3. Storz True Vista PMMA MIOL (Bausch & Lomb).

Pharmacia, have been manufacturing diffractive MIOLs. The Pharmacia Ceeon 811E (Monrovia, Calif) lens has been extensively implanted outside of the US.

Three-Zone Refractive MIOL

Concurrent with diffractive MIOL investigation, many other refractive designs were being studied. A variety of three-zone MIOLs, providing distance and near vision by using a near annulus at various distances from the central distance component, were manufactured by Alcon, Pharmacia, and Storz. The Storz True Vista has gained popularity, especially in European countries (Figure 16-3).

A multicenter European study reported by Knorz demonstrated excellent distance acuity (20/40 or better in 97%) with the True Vista, except at low contrast. Near acuity was satisfactory in 64%. Dr. Knorz found that this MIOL "emphasizes the far focus."[9,10] Shoji also evaluated the True Vista MIOL and found better near acuities with the P359-TUV model, reporting 79% obtaining J_1 or better near vision with distance correction only. He found that there was no significant difference in contrast sensitivity between multifocal and monofocal patients if the multifocal patients had bilateral MIOLs.[11]

Normal pupil patients can enjoy both near and distance vision, but smaller pupils tend to obstruct the near component with some three-zone MIOLs. However, smaller pupils may enhance contrast sensitivity. A study by Knorz and Koch demonstrated a loss of best-corrected contrast acuity with increasing pupillary size with the True Vista MIOL eyes and monofocal eyes, yet statistically greater with MIOL patients.[12] One advantage of this lens design is that even though there is pupil dependency, distance vision is always preserved despite the loss of near acuity due to miosis.

The Array MIOL

The Allergan Array multifocal IOL was the first MIOL to be granted premarket approval by the FDA, receiving this status in September of 1997. Over 100,000 Array MIOLs have been implanted, making the Array the most popular multifocal worldwide.

The optical composition of the Array has been termed "zonal progressive," a refractive design that incorporates five blended aspheric zones of power on the anterior sur-

Figure 16-4. Array silicone MIOL (Allergan).

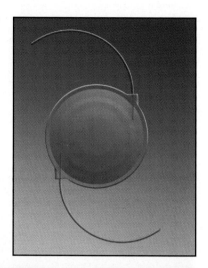

Figure 16-5. The central 2.1 mm of the optic is dedicated to distance vision, with the first near ring positioned from 2.1 mm to 3.4 mm, followed by a distance zone, then another near zone.

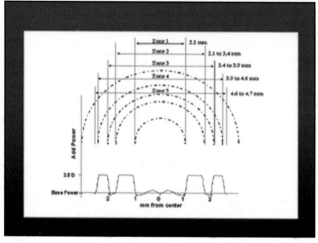

face of the optic (Figure 16-4). The central 2.1 mm of the optic is dedicated to distance vision, with the first near ring positioned from 2.1 mm to 3.4 mm, followed by a distance zone, then another near zone (Figure 16-5). The Array is considered a "distance dominant" MIOL with 50% of light transmission assigned to distance vision, 13% to intermediate, and 37% to near. With the current add power of 3.5 D (2.3 D effective power at the spectacle plane), near vision of at least J_3 is commonly seen, sometimes calling for an additional spectacle add with certain near vision requirements, such as very fine print. Like three-zone refractive MIOLs, the Array tends to lose a portion of its near function as the pupil becomes smaller than 2.0 mm.

The Array is currently only manufactured with a 6.0 mm silicone optic (plans are being made for an acrylic Array, a modification of the Sensar monofocal IOL). The ability to insert the foldable silicone SA40 Array through a small incision has been a real asset for this lens. Whether using folding forceps or the Allergan Unfolder, unwanted induced astigmatism is less likely to occur compared to rigid PMMA MIOLs.

During clinical trials before premarket approval, a number of new study methods were undertaken in order to demonstrate the relative benefits of the Array compared to monofocal IOLs. Traditionally, visual data and complication rates have been the major criteria for clinical evaluation of multifocal (and monofocal) IOLs. Array investigators employed a new concept, that of "quality of life" studies, to learn just how the multifocal vision that patients experience after Array implantation impacts their daily lives. Instead of just measuring visual acuity, quality of life assessment was used to measure visual function. In a multicenter, retrospective, randomized, clinical trial, the Array patients reported substantially higher quality of life ratings compared to monofocal controls, as reported by Javitt et al.[13]

Steinert led an earlier randomized, double-masked, multicenter trial to clinically evaluate the PMMA forerunner to the silicone Array, the Array MPC-25NB. The Array implanted eyes, as expected, were found to have some loss of low contrast acuity. Glare and light sensitivity ratings were similar between Array and monofocal controls. The cumulative patient survey results showed significantly greater patient satisfaction in the Array group.[14]

A more recent multicenter investigation carried out by a double-masked, prospective method yielded similar clinical results. Using the criteria of uncorrected distance vision of 20/40 or better combined with near vision of J_3 or better, 77% of eyes with the Array met the combined criteria, compared to 46% of eyes receiving the monofocal IOL. As with other MIOLs, loss of contrast sensitivity at low testing levels was statistically significant. Eyes with normal-sized resting pupils (2.5 to 4.0) exhibited 0.6 to 0.9 line reduction in Snellen acuity at low contrast levels. Statistically significant differences in symptom rating scores between Array patients and monofocal controls were observed at 1 year for reports of difficulty with halos (15% versus 6%), glare/flare (11% versus 12%), and blurred vision (4% versus 1%). In spite of these differences, patient satisfaction scores for Array patients were high (95% reported that they were moderately to very satisfied with their surgery).[15] The study protocol required surgeons to always aim for postoperative emmetropia in each eye. Therefore, postoperative monovision and/or intentional low postoperative astigmatism could not be employed to improve outcomes for monofocal eyes. This was necessary because the surgeon and clinical staff were unaware of which lens was to be implanted, the Array or the monofocal IOL. Therefore, tailoring the surgery to a specific IOL type was not possible.

An interesting subset in this study looked at the effect the Array had on driving ability. The thought was that driving evaluations may help to determine just what adverse consequences loss of contrast sensitivity and halos might produce. Bilaterally implanted Array patients and monofocal control patients were evaluated while behind the wheel of an automobile driving simulation unit at the University of Iowa. The driving performance of the patients participating in this study was evaluated with a variety of road and weather conditions, such as nighttime driving, night with glare, and fog. The results of this exercise showed that even though there were occasional situations in which monofocal patients did better (four of the 30 measures of performance), the multifocal patients still performed within the safety guidelines. This suggests that the level of reduction in low-contrast acuity and greater incidence of halos at night with the Array MIOL may not necessarily translate into poor visual function.

The Array represents the first real "proving ground" for MIOLs. As this multifocal lens continues to be successful, additional multifocal lens designs and enhancements of the Array lens are sure to follow. Since the Array FDA approval, a number of lessons have already been learned.

Patient satisfaction with MIOLs is most likely when:
1. Surgeons and clinical staff follow inclusion and exclusion criteria for patient selection.
2. Office systems are in place to improve IOL calculation accuracy.
3. Surgeons take advantage of the latest technology and techniques in cataract extraction.
4. Surgeons learn to reduce unwanted astigmatism.
5. Surgeons and their patients begin to regard poor uncorrected near vision after cataract surgery as an undesirable result.
6. Patients understand that, as with any new visual system, the process of visual cortical adaptation is necessary before optimal results are achieved.

REFERENCES

1. Keates R, Pearce J, Schneider R. Clinical results of the multifocal lens. *J Cataract Refract Surg.* 1987;13:557-560.
2. Ravalico G, Baccara F, Rinaldi G. Contrast sensitivity in multifocal intraocular lenses. *J Cataract Refract Surg.* 1993;19:22-25.
3. Wallace RB. *Current Concepts of Multifocal Intraocular Lenses.* Thorofare, NJ: SLACK Incorporated;1991.
4. Simpson MJ. The diffractive multifocal intraocular lens. *European J Implant Ref Surg.* 1989; 1:115-121.
5. Lindstrom R. Food and Drug Administration study update–one year results from 671 patients with the 3M multifocal intraocular lens. *Ophthalmology.* 1993;100:91-97.
6. Gimbel H, Sanders D, Raanan M. Visual and refractive results of multifocal intraocular lenses. *Ophthalmology.* 1991;98:881-888.
7. Auffarth G, Hunold W, Breitenbach S, et al. Long-term results for glare and contrast sensitivity in patients with diffractive, multifocal intraocular lenses. *European J Implant Ref Surg.* 1994;6:40-45.
8. Bellucci R, Giardini P. Pseudoaccommodation with the 3M diffractive multifocal intraocular lens: A refraction study of 52 subjects. *J Cataract Refract Surg.* 1993;19:32-35.
9. Knorz M. Results of the "True Vista" Bifocal IOL european multicentre study. *European J Implant Ref Surg.* 1992;4:245-248.
10. Knorz M, Aron-Rosa D, Claessens D, et al. Vision with the True Vista bifocal IOL. *European J Implant Ref Surg.* 1992;4:95-98.
11. Shoji N, Shimizu K. Clinical evaluation of a 5.5 mm three-zone refractive multifocal intraocular lens. *J Cataract Refract Surg.* 1996; 22:1097-1101.
12. Knorz M, Koch D, Martinez-Franco C, Lorger C. Effect of pupil size and astigmatism on contrast acuity with monofocal and bifocal intraocular lenses. *J Cataract Refract Surg.* 1994; 20:26-33.
13. Javitt JC, Wang F, Trentacost D, et al. Outcomes of cataract extraction with multifocal intraocular lens implantation. *Ophthalmology.* 1997;104:589-599.
14. Steinert R, Post C, Brint S, et al. A prospective, randomized, double-masked comparison of a zonal-progressive multifocal intraocular lens and a monofocal intraocular lens. *Ophthalmology.* 1992;99:853-860.
15. Steinert R, Aker B, Trentacost D, et al. A prospective comparative study of the AMO Array zonal-progressive multifocal silicone intraocular lens and a monofocal intraocular lens. *Ophthalmology.* 1999;106:1243-1255.

17

Patient Selection and Counseling for Multifocal IOL Insertion

Tom M. Coffman, MD
Philippe Dublineau, MD
I. Howard Fine, MD
Ivan Marais, MD
Kevin L. Waltz, MD

PATIENT SELECTION AND PATIENT COUNSELING

Tom M. Coffman, MD

The Array multifocal lens is a lens that is so exciting for cataract patients that the surgeon will generally gain an enormous amount of confidence very early. Generally, I believe most surgeons will use the Array in one or two patients a week initially. They will choose patients that have very little astigmatism or have astigmatism in the 0.5 D range, with the plus axis in the axis of their incision, and then watch their results. After the surgeon has performed 30 or 40 implants, he or she will certainly have gained a significant amount of confidence. In fact, my 40th patient was my mother-in-law, who had worn glasses since she was 24 and at 82 hasn't worn glasses since her Array lenses were implanted 2 years ago. Once the surgeon hits 500 to 1000 implants he realizes that he can predict results so closely and make patients so happy, that it doesn't make sense for presbyopic patients desiring LASIK, INTACS, or any other type of refractive surgery to have anything but the Array multifocal lens so that we can solve both problems: the necessity for glasses for distance and near by doing a clear lens exchange. Patient counseling pertains primarily to the possible postoperative nuisances such as glare or an off-center lens, although these occur in very small percentages. The information in this chapter was gleaned from my first 2000 Array implantations and hopefully will be helpful.

Patient Selection

The primary consideration for selecting good candidates for a multifocal Array lens is whether or not they are correctable to 20/30 or better postoperatively. This may be ascertained by evaluating the vision through the existing cataract and then looking at the macula to decide how much of the visual problem is due to the cataract and how much is due to any macular changes. If it appears that the patient should obtain 20/30 vision or better, I think that he is an excellent candidate for the Array lens.

If the patient has a monofocal implant in one eye and desires a multifocal in the second eye, one needs to explain that his eyes should match, and he should not have a multifocal lens in the second eye. However, as time has gone on, more and more surgeons have been implanting a monofocal in one eye and a multifocal in the other, and probably 98% of their patients are happy. For the 2% that do not like the differences between the two eyes, with a multifocal in one eye and a monofocal in the second eye, the patient might like either one better. Before any surgery, it needs to be discussed in detail that if he or she is unhappy with the imbalance, there are two options. One is to remove the multifocal and replace it with a monofocal, the other is to remove the monofocal and put in a multifocal. The latter would likely be at the patient's expense and not covered by insurance. The patient must understand up front that he or she has about a 2% chance of being unhappy and needing additional surgery to correct his or her imbalance.

If the patient has a significant cataract in one eye needing extraction and the second eye only has a moderate cataract, say with 20/40 vision that won't need surgery for some time, then the same type of process needs to be discussed.

I have performed about 150 Array implants in patients with a cataract in only one eye that was bad enough to require extraction. In these cases, I explained to the patient that if he or she is bothered postoperatively because of the difference in vision between the eyes, then we might take out the mild cataract sooner instead of later, or he or she would have the option to have the lens removed as a clear lens exchange at his or her expense. Of the 150 or so patients in whom I have performed the operation in just one eye, not one patient has been unhappy and asked that we do something with the second eye. Several dozen have been extremely happy and have asked to do the second eye so that they may enjoy the vision they experienced in the first eye with the Array lens.

A similar situation exists in patients who have over 2.0 D of anisometropia after achieving a monocular plano refractive error with the Array lens. In those cases, again I offer them the option of doing the second eye as a clear lens exchange at their expense to balance them if the anisometropia is unbearable. Rather than depriving these patients of the distance and near vision benefits of the Array lens by using a monofocal lens to avoid any of these situations, I prefer to offer these options in order that they might try the Array lens. Virtually every patient has been extremely happy.

Higher Level of Cataract Surgery

When surgeons decide to use the Array multifocal lens, they must understand that they are offering a higher level of cataract surgery to their patients. It is, in fact, refractive cataract surgery, which requires enormous attention to detail initially (quite beneficial to the surgeon's general operative technique). It is also helpful to use the Allergan SI40 platform, which is the same lens as the Array but without the multifocal front surface. This will establish the accuracy of the biometry being performed on the patients and the alterations in surgical technique. When the postoperative results are recorded and compared among the patients and the technicians doing the biometry, it becomes obvious if one of the technicians is better than another, and whether additional training may be needed for certain technicians.

It is certainly beneficial to perform an astigmatic keratotomy (or a corneal limbal relaxing incision) in all cataract surgery where the patient's astigmatism is over 1.0 to 1.5 D. These techniques are very simple and unlikely to cause any harm to the patients. It can be tried and perfected in patients receiving any type of implant.

Age

I feel the Array multifocal lens is the ideal lens for surgical corrections in pediatric cataract cases. The youngest patient I have implanted was 18 months of age. Children under 6 years need to be left hyperopic to grow into the distance part of their lens. In the past we have always had to fit them with hyperopic bifocals. Now, we may have to do that when they are very young. When the child is around 3 years old, the reading part of his or her prescription will actually function for distance vision since it is already 2.75 D less hyperopic than the distance prescription. So, even if the child is not wearing his or her glasses this would decrease the chance of amblyopia in that eye. Also since it is rather difficult to be exact with the prescription in children, if we are off by some value, we still have a 2.75 D range in the Array lens to get us by until the child is older. Hopefully this will help to alleviate amblyopia as well. I feel the Array is also an excellent lens for any patient under 40 because with a monofocal lens we would be unnecessarily committing them to presbyopia for a lifetime at an early age. Most cataracts in patients under 40 are the result of trauma, and therefore are usually only in one eye. Implanted, the Array lens makes the patient effectively normal. Not once have I seen one of these patients upset with the difference between one eye and the other.

For patients over 40 who have already experienced the major nuisance of presbyopia, the Array lens is a wonderful improvement for them. These are the happiest patients of all. In conclusion, I believe it is the ideal lens for most patients of any age.

Obsessive Compulsive Disorder

The patient with obsessive-compulsive disorder also deserve the best we can provide them. Therefore, I think they should have the Array multifocal lens unless there is some other contraindication. These patients are always difficult no matter what surgery they undergo. The best approach is to educate them at length as to the pros and cons and provide realistic postoperative expectations. Certainly, they will ask a lot of questions, but at least they will be more informed. I have had to remove one multifocal IOL from an obsessive-compulsive patient because of his disorder and not because of the implant. He developed cystoid macular edema (CME) and was sure it was the result of the new "fancy" implant and the fact that I had to piggyback the Array to a monofocal in order to give him his full correction.

Job or Hobby Requirements

With patients in whom very fine near vision is required, such as a watch maker or a jeweler, I always try to explain that they will likely need some slight reading magnification postoperatively to enable them to do the finest work. However, their general activities will often not require the magnifiers. One type of patient in whom I do not recommend the lens is a patient who drives at night for a living, such as a truck or limousine driver. Actually, 96% of them would probably do well, but I don't care to remove and replace the lens in the 0.5% to 4% who may develop nuisance-type problems. Reportedly, pilots really enjoy this lens because those in the presbyotic age group can see all the switches above their heads without throwing their heads back to look through their bifocals as they previously had to do. The only concern would be landing at night. However, glare coming from the landing lights would not likely be a significant problem. The main concern to the pilot would be whether the light is red or white, not whether there is flare coming from the light.

Clear Lens Exchange

Earlier, I alluded to the benefit for some patients of clear lens exchange in the second eye. However, as each surgeon becomes more satisfied with his predictable postoperative results, he will realize it is an excellent refractive procedure for all patients in the presbyopic age group. It is also, in my mind, the procedure of choice for myopes over −10.0 D as far as predictability and satisfactory postoperative results related to other options. This group must understand the approximately 2% increase in retinal detachment over their lifetime if their eyes are between 26 mm and 28 mm in axial length. They should also have a peripheral retinal examination preoperatively, postoperatively, and annually. Hyperopes of any level, and in particular over +3 D, love this lens and the visual results they obtain. The percentage of the population that are candidates for a clear lens exchange far exceeds the patients that are candidates for LASIK, INTACS, or whatever other current refractive procedure one might choose.

Results

Using the criteria that I have outlined above, I have performed the multifocal implant on 65% of my cataract surgery patients. The clear lens extraction is rapidly becoming a significant portion of my refractive practice. When I originally started doing the multifocal lens implant, I did it in only 6% of my patients within the first month, then 12% the next, 15 % the next, 25% the next, and so on until reaching my present 65% usage rate.

Patient Counseling

Time with the Patient

Initially, we are all concerned with this lens and what the patient might think about it postoperatively. We often spend a fair amount of time discussing the pros and cons of this lens with the first several patients. Eventually one realizes that the patients do not understand most of this discussion and confidence levels grow to the point where we likely do not spend any more time than we do with any other patient. We just discuss the different aspects of the multifocal to put them at ease.

Preoperative Discussion

When I have decided that a patient is ready for cataract surgery and that he or she will benefit most from the Array multifocal lens, I usually tell him or her that, "I feel I can improve your vision significantly by removing the cataract and I would like to use the new lens that may allow you to see distance and near without glasses much of the time." Sometimes I explain to them that 34% of my patients never wear glasses again postoperatively, and that 96% either never wear glasses again or just wear them occasionally, usually for small print or in dim light. I often ask the patient if he or she drives at night more than the average person. I mention that the down side of the lens is that there is a 4% chance that he or she will have enough bothersome night glare so that he or she won't care to drive at night. I also explain that I can prescribe different night time driving glasses, as well as an eyedrop that will usually reduce the patient's glare to the point that only 0.5% of patients with the Array would rather have somebody else drive at night than themselves. I feel that it is important for the patient to understand this because if he is in that 0.5%, he will be a bit disgruntled that he doesn't have quite the independence at night that he or she used to. My patients that have ended up in this 0.5% talk about it and are bothered by it; but only three of them have asked me to remove the lens and place a monofocal, therefore losing the ability to read without glasses most of the time.

When I finish this discussion I have a separate sheet of paper (Figure 17-1) discussing the night glare. I ask them to read and sign this form so that they have a copy and I have a copy in the chart to confirm they are aware of this one possible nuisance that they may experience. Sometimes preoperatively, I discuss the fact that postoperatively they may notice a ghost image on the edge of letters or objects. However, this tends to disappear over time and is due to the fact that they have two images in focus all of the time, one distance and one near, and one appears as a ghost some of the time. This is rarely a concern but has been noticed by some of my patients. I think it is important preoperatively to explain to the patient that if he or she is bothered by nighttime glare and ghost images, it is important to eliminate or reduce these images significantly by having the second eye done. It is certainly better to explain this to the patient preoperatively than to try to explain it postoperatively.

Postoperative Counseling

Since approximately 4% of Array patients may experience nighttime glare in a high-contrast situation such as a dark street, a single car with headlights or tail lights, or a street light, the possible solutions to this problem need to be addressed.

As explained before, the most successful way to reduce glare is to perform the multi-focal in the second eye. Also, if the posterior capsule becomes somewhat thickened or even mildly hazy to the 20/25 level, it needs to be lasered. A posterior capsulotomy can significantly improve the near vision, and sometimes the distance vision, and can decrease some of the glare. If the patient requires any residual postoperative glasses correction, I would give him or her corrective lenses for nighttime driving. If, however, the prescription is near plano, or if the normal distance prescription does not work, I would prescribe a distance prescription with an additional -7.50 in order to make the patient mildly hyperopic. The glare is moderately reduced in mild hyperopia as opposed to mild myopia. In that pair of glasses I would also consider polarization with the smallest amount of tint (in the 5% to 10% range). I have not found polarization to be particularly effective, and it can cost $100.00 per pair of glasses. However, I often give these patients the option. In some patients, either before or after trying the glasses, one might try 0.5% pilocarpine in each eye at sundown. In some patients, this is only required in one eye to significantly reduce the nighttime glare. Patients must be warned of the brow ache they may experience during the first week or two of use.

Lens Centration

If the glare increases, the vision decreases, or if the cylinder changes, the implant may have moved off center. Usually 0.5 mm of decentration is not significant. However, somewhere around 0.75 to 1.0 mm off center can become important to a patient's vision and create more glare.

The most common cause of decentration results from the anterior/posterior capsular scarring pushing or pulling the lens off center. Recentration of the lens is usually rather easy. The procedure generally takes about 1 minute and is performed in the operating

Important information you should be aware of when choosing the Multifocal Implant for your surgery.

You may be a candidate to receive a unique type of implant lens at the time of your cataract surgery. It is called the Multifocal Lens. This lens will be inserted into your eye much the same way as the conventional implant lenses that have been available for years. This newer style of implant has the potential to give those who receive it the ability to see objects clearly at distance and near without the need for glasses. Most of these people become much less dependent on glasses after surgery if they receive this lens, however glasses may still be required some of the time to provide optimal vision for some patients. A small percentage of the patients who received this lens in the past have experienced glare while looking towards lights at night. This glare has been known to hinder some patient's ability to drive a vehicle comfortably at night.

I understand that there is no guarantee that I will never have to wear glasses again, although it is believed that my dependency on glasses will be greatly decreased.

Patient Name (print)_____

Patient Signature_____ Date_____

Physicians Signature_____ Date_____

Figure 17-1. Night glare disclosure form.

room where I have all the necessary equipment in a sterile environment. I make a side-port incision at 2:30 and at 9:30 o'clock, and usually inject 1% preservative-free Xylocaine (Astra USA Inc, Westboro, Mass) in the dilated eye. I then use a Sinsky hook to rotate the lens to a more centered position, keeping the lens in the bag if possible. A significant exception to this is if the patient ended up with low hyperopia in the vicinity of +0.75 D. In this situation, I would rotate the lens from the bag into the sulcus. This maneuver will correct the refractive error as well as recenter the lens. If the lens is rotated into the sulcus, it has only a 50% chance of staying centered in the sulcus if this repositioning is performed over a week after the initial procedure. Obviously, it is always preferable to try to keep the haptics in the bag for long-term lens centration.

Coffman Haptic Expansion Technique

If at some point the lens will not stay centered in the bag or the sulcus, I have devised a technique to expand the haptics so that the lens will stay better centered. I make the two side-port incisions as I mentioned before, at 2:30 and 9:30 o'clock, making them slightly larger than needed for a Sinsky hook. In fact, make them large enough for a Kuglen, h-shaped hook. I then inject some viscoelastic anterior to the lens. I can then put one Kuglen hook through each incision, placing one of the hooks at a haptic lens junction. I put counter force with the second hook on the inside of the loop adjacent to the first hook and bend it backward to the point that it does not come back to its original position, which then makes the loop fit a much larger diameter.

This can be done in the bag, in the sulcus, or even in the AC. Sometimes the lens will stay in place and make it easy. Other times it will want to spin and will have to be pushed to one side or the other until it holds sufficiently to bend the haptic. Once this is performed on each haptic, I then spin the lens until I find a place in the bag or sulcus where the lens stays centered even when challenged by BSS reinflation and/or nudging with the BSS cannula. Usually these two side-port incisions don't seal easily. Stromal hydration of these incisions may be needed to maintain the anterior chamber pressure. In those cases in which viscoelastic is required to maintain the anterior chamber, it is best to wash out the remaining viscoelastic with BSS through a large cannula at the end of the case.

Micromonovision

When the postoperative refraction in any patient is +0.25 D or greater and his or her distance vision is good but his or her near vision is not 20/30 or better, I prefer to place an Array lens in the second eye, which will result in a -0.25 postoperative result. This will give the patient a good range of focus with both eyes open for distance and near vision.

Small Pupils

For Array patients who have small pupils and, as a result, have early difficulty, I recommend waiting at least 3 to 6 months. I explain that his or her near vision will improve on its own as he or she gets used to using these fancy new lenses. At some point, I might consider trying 2.5% Neosynpherine. If this helps, maybe an argon laser pupilloplasty might be a solution. This procedure enlarges the pupil and may give the patient better near vision.

The one possible down side to pupil enlargement would be the possibility of increasing night glare, which needs to be discussed with the patient. Possibly the use of Neosynephrine drops will let the patient and the surgeon know ahead of time whether or not the pupilloplasty should be performed. The pupilloplasty is done with a larger spot size and a lower power than usual just to heat up the iris 1 or 2 mm from the sphincter, shrinking the iris fibers and enlarging the pupillary aperture.

Remove and Replace the Multifocal

If a patient cannot physically tolerate the glare or has a personality that cannot tolerate the glare, then sometimes it is better to replace the multifocal IOL with an SI40 monofocal lens. This has only occurred in three eyes in my first 2000 multifocal implants. Since it takes so many months to try all of the possible solutions to alleviate glare, it will be highly unlikely that the new lens can be implanted in the capsular bag. Fortunately, the SI40 works quite well in the sulcus in most patients. For those few in whom it will not center, the Coffman haptic expansion technique may be required. When calculating the lens power, it is helpful to use the refraction for the existing Array lens (unless it is so far off center you are refracting the near part of the lens). If at some point the lens was centered and you have a good refraction, that would be helpful. One must take into account that when the lens is placed in the sulcus instead of the bag, about 0.5 D less power of the capsular lens is needed to achieve the same refractive result. Occasionally, moving the lens from bag to the sulcus makes the eye a whole diopter more myopic, but that is rare.

To pick the new lens power, I would compare the most accurate prescription I have and then run the original calculations again for placement in the sulcus, or just use the original calculation for placement in the bag and subtract 0.5 D of power if the eye was near plano. To remove the lens, I usually go through the old incision unless I cannot open it with a Sinsky hook, in which case I just make a new incision. The opening needs to be approximately 4 mm wide to remove the old lens, which is most easily removed by spinning the lens out of the bag. This is done by placing the Sinsky hook in the crotch of the lens-haptic junction and pulling or pushing so that it is dialed out of the tube encasing the haptic. This is not difficult and does not offer much resistance. Getting the Sinsky hook into the bag in the postoperative eye, especially with capsular phimosis, can be difficult. Once the lens is dialed into the anterior chamber, I tease one haptic out of the eye and, while grasping it with tying forceps under viscoelastic, I often grasp the optic with Shepherd forceps that we once used for PMMA lenses years ago. Another method is to take two toothed forceps and pull the lens hand-over-hand until it comes out of the eye, which is quite easily done through a 4 mm opening. When the new monofocal lens is put into the sulcus, it is important to rotate it into a position so that when challenged with BSS inflation or a cannula, the lens stays in a central position.

Counseling Clear Lens Exchange Patients

One of the first things I noticed when I started to do clear lens exchanges was that often the patients ended up 0.75 to 1.0 D hyperopic.

The sound waves for the A-scan go through a clear lens at a different speed than a cataract lens; even though this is taken into account, there is likely little background data for past clear lens exchange formulas to make them as accurate as we would like them to be. Therefore, I always aim for -0.50 D for clear lens exchange patients to have a better chance of ending up with a plano prescription postoperatively. If I do end up with a +0.75 to 1.0 D result postoperatively at the end of 1 week, the following day I will dial that lens from the bag into the sulcus, correcting the problem in most patients as long as I can get it to center. This is usually not difficult at the end of 1 week, but at the end of 2 weeks, it can become difficult due to the loss of the elastic memory of the haptics. If one encounters the unfortunate result of a patient ending up -1.0 D after a clear lens exchange, I would do a single incision RK with a 5 mm optical zone and place the incision somewhere superiorly, or if there is any cylinder, in the meridian of the plus axis. If a patient had enough residual cylinder that he or she was unhappy with his or her visual result I would not hesitate to perform an astigmatic keratotomy. Generally the AK I perform at the time of the original surgery or postoperative is in at the 7 mm optical zone. I portion two incisions in the plus axis, 1 mm in length for each diopter of required correction with a minimum incision length of 1.5 mm and a maximum incision of 3.0 mm. When the AK is required in the axis of the incision for phacoemulsification, I place it opposite the phaco incision and use the same criteria for one incision that I do for two. If later on it is required to correct persistent cylinder in this meridian, I would make a second astigmatic keratotomy incision opposite from the first incision at the 7 mm optical zone and nearest to the original incision from the lens extraction.

As one can tell from this description of careful fine-tuning for the clear lens exchange, these patients often expect absolutely perfect results because they are paying you to get rid of their glasses. They are certainly the most difficult patients and are paying for that privilege. I usually explain to them preoperatively that to make them perfect I may go back at 1 week, 3 months, 6 months, or even later to make small enhancing modifications to their surgery. I also explain that most of these enhancing techniques take about 1 minute but require the use of the operating facility.

Happy Patients

The Array multifocal lens certainly has resulted in many happy postoperative patients. As we all know, most of our patients are referred to us by other happy patients. After I had initially used the Array for a few months and became very happy with the results, I did market the lens to some degree, which resulted in a 30% increase in my surgical volume over the ensuing few months. Without any additional advertising, my surgical volume increased over 10% over the entire first year. Most surgeons using the Array lens are amazed at the patient's "matter of fact" response to this lens. They expect to go without glasses most of the time and when that occurs, they consider it normal. The majority of the patients are happy with it, but just seem to expect their excellent visual results. Even with this attitude, the 10% increase in my practice was a significant change.

Associate Counseling

On a day-to-day basis, I see extremely happy recipients of the Array multifocal lens. My associates, however, only hear about the few patients that are upset with the glare. Therefore, I found it important to continually educate my associates as to the enormous percentage of happy patients. They must be reminded that 95% of my patients are 20/40 uncorrected distance and near and that only 4% of the patients have the glare that is disturbing to them. I must also emphasize to them that the 4% is reducible to about 0.5% with eye glasses and eyedrop techniques.

Conclusions

I feel that the Array multifocal lens is definitely the next higher level of cataract surgery. It is refractive cataract surgery and requires us all to pay more attention to detail and precise reproducible postoperative results. I have been extremely happy with the results in my first 2000 multifocal lenses implanted and, in fact, at this point feel very sorry for a patient who is not a candidate or for some reason does not receive a multifocal lens when a cataract extraction is indicated.

MY EXPERIENCE WITH MULTIFOCAL IOLS

PHILIPPE DUBLINEAU, MD

Since 1988, I have implanted more than 2600 multifocal lenses. In the first year, I implanted multifocal lenses in more than 50% of patients, falling to approximately 12% in the 3 years following. Since 1993, I have selected less than 15% of my patients for multifocal lens implantation.

Why has my use of multifocal lenses become less frequent? When multifocal lenses were first proposed, medical indications were not completely understood, because expectations were based on predictions provided by experiments with the optical bench. Unfortunately, the optical bench could not predict the problems that could arise after surgery and from incorrect patient selection. For example, in 1990, a 1.25 D induced astigmatism could be considered an acceptable result, while now this is a relative contraindication for the multifocal implant. Moreover, at that time we were not certain that emmetropia would be the best postoperative result.

Possibly, poor brain plasticity of our patients was the cause for bad results. In addition, our surgical techniques and the 6 mm diameter of the PMMA lens were not the best format for this new technology. Also, medical indications and contraindications for a cataract refractive procedure were not clearly defined. I eventually learned how important patient selection can be after witnessing the variable behavior early postoperative patients would exhibit when first experiencing simultaneous multifocal vision. With time, I have found that the slogan "less spectacles with MIOLs" is more accurate than "no spectacles with MIOLs."

Expanding the indications for multifocal lens use might begin to include patients that require more frequent use of glasses. These patients might be better candidates for monofocal IOLs. Additionally, being able to predict emmetropia as a means to diminish the necessity to wear glasses is critical to successful multifocal lens implantation. Therefore, the optimum use of multifocal IOLs may be no more than 15% to 18%. However, possible future improvements in clinical practice and IOL precision may permit an increase in their use.

My experience with multifocals has involved a variety of diffractive and refractive styles:

- 1200 diffractive 6 mm optic diameter, PMMA lenses with a 3.5 D add (3M Healthcare).
- 150 diffractive 6 mm optic diameter PMMA lenses with a 4.0 D add (Alcon Surgical).
- 775 multizonal 6 mm optic diameter, silicone lenses with a 3.5 D add with a central distance zone (Allergan).
- 84 refractive aspheric progressive 5.5 mm diameter, PMMA lenses with a 4.75 D add and a central near zone (Domilens and Bausch & Lomb Surgical).
- 191 refractive three zones, 5.5 mm diameter, PMMA lenses with a 4.0 D add and a central distance zone (Storz and Bausch & Lomb).
- 126 refractive four zones, 6 mm diameter, PMMA lenses, and 65 hydrophilic acrylic lenses with a 4.0 D add and a central near zone (Corneal).
- 74 refractive four zones, 6 mm diameter, hydrophilic acrylic lenses with a 4.0 D add and a central near zone (IOLTECH).

A universal multifocal implant does not exist. Each implant I have used represents a compromise between the near, intermediate, and distance vision.

The privilegiate vision is assessed by the optical engineers who have determined the percentage of light transmitted by various multifocal IOLs for various focal points in relation to the pupil diameter. All these lenses behave differently. Therefore, it is impossible to know which is the best multifocal implant for each patient.

It is necessary to select from the different technologies and from the different objectives of each lens as to which is best suited to the requirements of a specific patient.

In another way, the choice of the surgeon depends on his or her own philosophy and experience. Which lens would be the best choice?

- A very distance-dominant multifocal lens with a functional near vision that needs spectacles for near vision in two thirds of cases?
- A very near dominant multifocal lens with the distance vision that cannot be better than 20/30 most of time?
- A very intermediate dominant multifocal lens that frequently requires an additional add of +1.50 D for precise near vision?
- A good compromise between distance and near vision, such as a diffractive lens that causes less contrast sensitivity and more halos?

For beginning multifocal surgeons, I think the multizonal lens (Allergan) is preferable. It will provide distance vision as good as a monofocal IOL in daily life, and any necessary improvement in near vision can be produced by the occasional use of spectacles.

As soon as surgeons are convinced of the benefits of multifocal IOLs they will seek to obtain better near visual acuity without glasses, which is my personal objective.

In my experience, diffractive multifocal IOLs with a 4 D add (Alcon) have consistently produced the best results for universal distance and near vision, followed by the refractive implants of Storz. However, these implants were produced in rigid PMMA and tend to induce more astigmatism than foldable implants. In conclusion, I think that multifocal lenses are part of refractive surgery with a trend to an increasing market. These implants must give patients perfect near vision and good distance vision without halos while driving at night.

As for patient selection, there are ocular, refractive, socioprofessional, and general aspects that need to be considered regarding the patient.

Ocular Indications

- No other pathology other than cataract.
- Satisfactory quality of the postoperative tear film on which the good transparency of the cornea depends.
- The curve of the cornea must be regular, without defects in the visual axis. All corneal dystrophy patients should be eliminated.
- The pupil shape should be normal because there is a direct relationship between pupil diameter and the percentage of light transmission with refractive lenses. I eliminate patients with either too large or too small a pupil.
- A normal macula should be present with a perfect fovea without any drusen. Good vascularization of the optic nerve is also important.

Refractive Indications

- The astigmatism must be less than 1.0 D with-the-rule and 0.5 D against-the-rule for a temporal clear corneal incision.
- Because the postoperative results obtained after astigmatism surgery do not always correspond to the expectations of surgeons, I consider it best to select patients without astigmatism.
- Biometric results must be balanced between the two eyes and correspond to the power of the spectacles worn by the patient. Surgeons must have in mind one objective, emmetropia. Therefore, we must have confidence in the exact power of the lens needed for emmetropia predicted by preoperative biometry.

Socioprofessional Indications

- The occasional side effects produced by simultaneous multifocal vision, that of low contrast blurred vision and halos during night driving, must be taken into consideration.
- It is best to discourage professional or enthusiastic night drivers and patients who work in conditions of fluctuating light intensity.
- I carefully consider the personal visual habits of the patient in order to choose whether to implant a distance or near vision dominant multifocal lens.

General Status Indications

- Multifocal lenses are part of refractive surgery. We must try to eliminate worried, meticulous, or demanding patients.
- Due to problems caused by simultaneous multifocal vision, patients suffering from diseases producing a modification of behavior or diminishing contrast sensitivity should be avoided.

Patient Counseling

Even though multifocal lenses provide both near and distance vision, there is a probability of some important side effects. Patients who have been good candidates for MIOL implantation must be clearly advised of the advantages and disadvantages of these IOLs.

Advantages

- Multifocal lenses reduce the necessity to wear glasses in daily life, but glasses may be required for specific occasions, such as precise near and distance vision. It must be clear to patients that multifocal IOLs do not entirely obviate the necessity for glasses. According to my statistics, only 30% of patients never wear glasses.
- Patients are free of constraints in that they have the choice of wearing glasses or not.
- For near vision, the depth of focus of MIOLs enables the patient to read easily over a greater distance than with a monofocal lens.

Disadvantages

- The only real problem with multifocal lenses is halos at night, particularly when driving. Low-contrast conditions inevitably induce halos, and this factor must be made clear to patients. Psychologically, halos are not a concern for all patients. Some regard them simply as a slight inconvenience, while other patients are unaware of their existence.
- Loss of contrast sensitivity (this is less of a problem with photopic vision than in mesopic vision and diminishes with time).
- In daily life, at the worst, there will be a loss of up to two lines of vision when eyes are measured separately, but binocular vision will be less affected.

For those patients who complain of halos, I refuse a lens exchange because the halos diminish in 2 to 4 months, and the advantages that multifocal IOLs provide these patients generally outweigh the disadvantages.

PATIENT SELECTION

I. HOWARD FINE, MD

Our utilization of the Array multifocal IOL over the past 2 1/2 years has been extensive. We have implanted this lens in approximately 30% of our cataract patients, and in the majority of our clear lens replacement refractive surgery patients. As a result of our experience, we have developed specific guidelines with respect to the selection of candidates and surgical strategies that enhance outcomes with this IOL.

Allergan recommends using the Array multifocal IOL for bilateral cataract patients whose surgery is uncomplicated and whose personality is such that they are not likely to fixate on the presence of minor visual aberrations, such as halos around lights. There is obviously a broad range of patients who would be acceptable candidates. Relative or absolute contraindications include the presence of ocular pathologies other than cataracts that may degrade image formation or may be associated with less than adequate visual function postoperatively despite visual improvement following surgery. Pre-existing ocular pathologies that are frequently looked upon as contraindications include age-related macular degeneration, uncontrolled diabetes or diabetic retinopathy, uncontrolled glaucoma, recurrent inflammatory eye disease, retinal detachment risk, corneal disease, or previous refractive surgery in the form of radial keratotomy, photorefractive keratectomy, or laser assisted in-situ keratomileusis.

We avoid the utilization of these lenses in patients who complain excessively, are highly introspective and fussy, or obsess over body image and symptoms. We are conservative when evaluating patients with occupations that include frequent night driving and occupations that put high demands on vision and near work, such as engineers and architects. Such patients need to demonstrate a strong desire for relative spectacle independence in order to be considered for Array implantation.

In our practice, we have reduced patient selection to a very rapid process. Once we determine that someone is a candidate for either cataract extraction or clear lens replacement, we ask the patient two questions. The first question is, "If we could put an implant in your eye that would allow you to see both distance and near without glasses under most circumstances would that be an advantage?" Approximately 50% of our patients say "no" in one way or another. Those negative responses may include, "I don't mind wearing glasses," "My grandchildren wouldn't recognize me without glasses," "I look terrible without glasses," or "I've worn glasses all my life". These patients receive monofocal IOLs. For the 50% who say it would be an advantage, we ask a second question: "If the lens is associated with halos around lights at night, would it still be an advantage?" Approximately 60% of this group of patients say that they do not think they would be bothered by these symptoms, and they receive a multifocal IOL.

There are special circumstances in which implantation of a multifocal IOL should be strongly considered. Alzheimers patients frequently lose or misplace their spectacles and, thus, might benefit from the full range of view that a multifocal IOL provides without spectacles. Patients with arthritis of the neck or other conditions with limited range of motion of the neck may benefit from a multifocal IOL rather than multifocal spectacles that require changes in head position. Patients with a monocular cataract who have successfully worn monovision contact lenses should be considered possible candidates for monocular implantation. The same is true for certain occupations, such as photographers, who want to alternate focusing through the camera and adjust imaging parameters on the camera without wearing spectacles. In these patients, the focusing eye could have a monofocal IOL and the nondominant eye a multifocal. We almost always use the Array in traumatic cataracts in young adults in order to facilitate binocularity at near, especially if the fellow eye has no refractive error or is corrected by contact lenses.

Prior to implanting an Array, we inform all candidates of the lens' statistics reported in a recent study to ensure that they understand that spectacle independence is not guaranteed.[1] Approximately 41% of the patients implanted with bilateral Array IOLs in this study never needed to wear glasses, 50% wore glasses on a limited basis, such as driving at night or during prolonged reading, 12% always needed to wear glasses for near work, and approximately 8% needed to wear spectacles on a full-time basis for distance and near correction. In addition, 15% of patients were found to have difficulty with halos at night and 11% had difficulty with glare, compared to 6% and 1% respectively in monofocal patients.

UTILIZATION OF MULTIFOCAL IOLS

Ivan Marais, MD

In my practice, I have learned from experience that there are certain categories of patients who do well with multifocal IOLs. However, not every patient in these categories is suitable, and final selection will depend on the history, examination, and how he or she responds to counseling.

The benefits from multifocal IOLs are less spectacle dependency and a full range of vision. Numerous studies have shown that a large percentage of these patients never use spectacles and those that do only use them at times and for certain activities. The patients that need spectacles most of the time are usually those who have more than 1.25 D astigmatism or where there is a large biometric error.

Some degree of bifocality can be achieved with monofocal IOLs by monovision, making one eye myopic (about –1.5 D) and the other eye emmetropic or with astigmatism (preferably +0.75 sph –1.00 cyl axis 90° or 180°). However, in a comparative study of 50 bilateral multifocal implants and 50 carefully chosen monofocal patients who had achieved some degree of bifocality, the multifocal group performed far better in a wide range of activities.

The positive categories are:

- Patients who do not like wearing spectacles and want to be as spectacle independent as possible.
- Patients requesting multifocal implants, having heard of this technology by word of mouth.
- Hyperopia. These patients are usually totally spectacle dependent after the age of 50, especially those who are more than +1.50 D hyperopic. They are very grateful to have some spectacle independency and a full range of focus again postoperatively.
- Young unilateral cataracts patients. These cataracts are usually traumatic in origin. It is important to explain to these patients that with an IOL it is impossible to reproduce the tremendous accommodative powers a young person has, but it does enable them to see near and far without glasses. These patients tend to close one eye at a time after surgery to compare vision, and that will certainly make them unhappy. It must be stressed that the best vision is obtained by using both eyes

together, and they must stop making comparisons. Young bilateral cataract patients are also very suitable for multifocal implantation, provided there is no amblyopia.

- Certain occupations. In some occupations, a range of vision is required that can be achieved by wearing multifocal spectacles postoperatively; but with spectacles, the focus is dependent on head posture, which is not the case with multifocal IOLs. A range of vision without changing head posture is important in many occupations, such as a motor mechanic working under a car, professional musicians such as violinists, librarians, gastroenterologists using endoscopes, etc. I have done multifocal implants on many of these patients, including a commercial airline pilot, with very satisfying results. An American ophthalmologist has had multifocal implants and has no problem with any aspect of his profession, including microscopic surgery.
- Sport. Bilateral multifocal implant patients do very well in a variety of sports in which a range of focus is required. Notably shooting sports, snooker, tennis, golf, etc.
- Unilateral cataracts in presbyopes. Awareness of rings around lights is more pronounced in unilateral multifocal implants and improves after the fellow eye is implanted. However, unilateral multifocal implant patients have not, in my experience, been more aware of rings to a worrying degree. The surgery is very important to control this. There must be no induced astigmatism or myopia, no decentration or tilt, and normal pupillary action. Patient selection criteria is similar to bilateral implants, but only those patients are chosen that definitely want to have the multifocal range. Hyperopic patients particularly like this technology and frequently beg for clear lensectomy in the fellow eye once they have compared the two eyes. I have also found that in cases in which the unoperated eye is slightly myopic, there is much less spectacle dependency postoperatively because near vision is enhanced. Some of the patients that fall into these categories may, however, not be suitable and that is determined by taking a history and doing an examination.

Exclusion Criteria

History

- Habitual spectacle wearers feel undressed without them.
- Patients that are very light sensitive and are dazzled by lights of oncoming cars at night, even before the cataracts started.
- Patients that are very apprehensive after mentioning rings around lights and wonder if they could handle it.
- Ultra finicky patients that bring you diagrams of their vitreous floaters and have unrealistic expectations. These patients will always complain and find fault with everything (fortunately, all of these categories of patients are rare).

Examination

Cornea

- Any corneal pathology that affects vision.
- Corneal scars that cause light scattering.

- Irregular astigmatism.
- Regular astigmatism greater than 1.25 D unless it is corrected.

In my opinion, it is essential to keep astigmatism to 0.75 D or less to fully utilize multifocal technology. In fact, if a –0.75 D cylinder placed in front of the eye makes a significant difference to vision binocularly, I do a mini AK to correct this.

My surgical preference is a 2.8 mm clear cornea, temporal approach incision that does not induce astigmatism. Three quarters to 2.00 D is treated with curvilinear T cuts in a 7 mm optic zone, and greater than 2.00 D with the Canrobert markers. The cuts can either be made freehand, or more accurately, with the Mastell pivotal diamond knife system. I have been doing these astigmatic corrective procedures for many years and have not found any visual aberrations as a result of these incisions.

Iris and Pupil

- Sector iridectomy.
- Fixed dilated pupil.
- Miosis with very poor dilatation.

These cases are generally not suitable. The first two would result in accentuation of the rings around lights, flares, and edge glare. The miosis would result in difficulty in utilizing the reading adds. However, if a patient with any of these problems would definitely benefit from a multifocal IOL, it can still work with modified techniques.

For the iridectomy or dilated pupil, a 4 mm capsulorrhexis is made in the center of the optic zone. All the lens matter is removed with great care to prevent capsular contraction, but the capsule is not polished. The anterior capsule will opacify leaving a 4 mm pupil. With the miosis, the pupil can be stretched or partial sphincterotomy cuts made.

Lens

- Subluxated lenses.
- Post vitrectomy.

These cases can be suitable for multifocal implantation after the insertion of a capsular tension ring; and it may sometimes be necessary to insert a transcleral suture to secure the superior haptic and thus center the lens.

Retina

- Excluded are cases with retinal problems, such as bad diabetics with proliferative retinopathy or cases that may require silicone oil.
- Retinal detachments and membrane stripping do not seem to present any problems to retinal surgeons after multifocal implantation.

Macular Degeneration

- In dry atrophy, patients do benefit from the multifocal IOL by having two reading additions. One is using the distance part of the IOL plus the spectacle add, and two is using the near part of the IOL plus the spectacle add. The latter is for smaller print, while there is still some macular function left.
- With no central vision, the multifocal is not indicated.

Lens Power Not Available

Some surgeons have solved this problem by doing piggybacks, putting the multifocal in the ciliary sulcus and the other lens in the bag.

Counseling

- It is important not to promise too much. If the patients are promised they will get perfect near, intermediate, and distance vision, they will be disappointed. I only tell them that they will be less spectacle dependent. If they never need glasses, it will be a pleasant surprise.
- I do not mention that there will be some loss of contrast, because nobody ever notices it.
- Adaptation. Some patients do not adapt immediately, but their reading ability may improve after a week or so. I try to delay prescribing reading glasses as long as possible.
- Halos. These are defocused rings around lights and I play these down as much as possible. The more fuss there is made about them, the more patients will be aware of them. For the few patients for whom night driving is a real problem, it is important to reassure them. They usually improve after a few months, and especially so when the second eye is done. In very rare cases, I prescribe 0.5% or 1% pilocarpine drops to be inserted 15 minutes before driving and I find they need this less and less as time goes by. Tinting of the upper part of spectacles or prescribing of -1.50 dioptic spheres also helps. During counseling, my patients are told there will be rings around lights, but they will not be noticed after a short while. The rings are essential because that is how multifocality comes about.
- It is stressed that even with monofocal lenses there are flares. During the day, no rings or flares are noticed. We have omitted telling a few patients about the rings and most of these never complained about it.

IOL Designs

An IOL with more than one focus can be either a bifocal or a multifocal. My own preference is for a multifocal because this gives a range of vision and not just near and distance corrections.

To achieve this, there must be a progressive element (in other words, a gradual transition of power that gives a range of vision). With abrupt power changes, there is a scattering of light, which is the case with bifocals. Pure progressive lenses are also no good because light is spread equally over the whole range and no focal point is absolutely clear. The answer, therefore, is to have zones with gradual, progressive power changes between them. The central zone, which would be the dominant zone, should be for distance, and most light will then be used for distance. The number of zones is important, as it has been shown that pupil size has less effect with five zones than with three. In my opinion, a five zonal progressive IOL is the best design.

It would be interesting to see if the central zone of the IOL was made for near in the nondominant eye, whether this would improve the overall vision.

Advice for Surgeons Starting With Multifocal IOLs

Biometry

It is important that the surgeon does accurate biometry. To do this, the IOL must always be placed in the bag, preferably with a rim of anterior capsule covering the edges of the lens all round. This prevents the optic from popping out of the bag with a resultant myopic shift. It also prevents tilting and reduces posterior capsular opacification. The biometry is aimed at emmetropia, and if there is an error, to err on the plus side. Erring on the minus side accentuates the rings around lights, and spectacles may therefore be necessary for distance vision. It also brings the near focus closer.

Astigmatism

This must be controlled, therefore, the phaco incision must not be greater than 3.2 mm.

Patient Selection

Choose a very easy cataract with a soft nucleus and a healthy retina. The anterior chamber depth must be normal and the pupil must dilate well. The patient must want to be as spectacle independent as possible and must not be put off by the question of rings around lights.

With more experience, the surgeon can extend the selection criteria.

Counseling

Do not promise too much and play down the rings around lights. Mention adaptation and perhaps that if worse came to worse, the IOL can be replaced with a monofocal. I have personally never explanted a multifocal IOL in 1200 cases.

MY PERSONAL EXPERIENCE WITH THE ARRAY
N̶   ̶I̶O̶L̶

Make this your last sticky...

I have been implanting Arra   een a bilateral Array patient myself for 20 mo   :perience first- hand the benefits of being a mu   patients on the benefits and drawbacks of the   atient benefits to having a multifocal IOL and   be understood by both the doctor and the pa   pective of hav- ing been simultaneously on bc

Background

I was the first ophthalmolo   d with the Array multifocal IOL. I was willing t   enced all of the alternatives. I was 13 years o   y were approxi- mately –2.00 D with a little c   he form of a flat

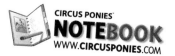

top 25 mm segment. I had a high accommodative convergence/accommodation (AC/A) ratio with a high esophoria. I was being treated by a "functional" optometrist to decrease my visual strain at near.

The concept worked well for me and I wore essentially the same prescription—glasses with bifocals—for the next 23 years. I wore them through all of high school, college, optometry school, optometry fellowship, medical school, internship, ophthalmology residency, and oculoplastic fellowship. I had no concept of what it was like to see without glasses at distance and bifocals at near. Although I was not a presbyope, I had over two decades of bifocal experience by the time I was 36 years old.

I was driving on a highway during the last several months of my oculoplastic fellowship in the spring of 1992 when I became irritated with how poorly I was able to see with my glasses. I took them off to clean them. I was shocked to discover I could see great without my glasses for the first time in my memory. I was 20/20+ without correction in each eye! It was an incredible feeling. I was elated and scared. I was scared something dreadful was going to happen because it was so unnatural to spontaneously resolve 2.00 diopters of myopia without a laser. I had two separate eye examinations, without telling anyone why, and I was pronounced normal.

I had experienced a miracle of such an incredible magnitude that it would take 8 more years for me to understand it. Several years later, after I was diagnosed with cataracts, I would learn that my mother's side of the family had a history of early cataracts. The cataracts tended to occur about 5 to 10 years after an approximately 2.00 D refractive shift toward hyperopia. My mother had successful cataract surgery in the mid 1980s with a monofocal PMMA IOL.

I enjoyed 5 years of fantastic vision without glasses coinciding with the first 5 years of surgical practice after my oculoplastic fellowship. These 5 years of emmetropia without presbyopia, preceded by the 23 years of bifocals, were the foundation for my willingness to be the first ophthalmologist to be bilaterally implanted with the Array multifocal IOL. By several quirks of fate, I had tried the alternatives and I was willing to take a risk to get what I wanted—life-long freedom from glasses.

My Diagnostic Experience

During 1997 I experienced intermittent bouts of poor visual quality. I attributed it to my long-term dry eye syndrome. I used artificial tears with increasing frequency and decreasing effectiveness. I repeatedly checked to see if I was developing a new refractive error, but I was not. I had my eyes examined with a slit lamp early in 1997 to confirm the dry eyes, and no cataract was seen. By January 1998, the symptoms had become quite distressing.

I was having severe difficulty with glare, especially driving at night. I was seeing floaters regularly when using an operating microscope. I was sure my reading speed was dropping, and I believed my reading comprehension was decreasing. I was 41 years old and I wondered if this was the beginning of old age. The possibility of cataracts was not even considered; I was an ophthalmic microsurgeon. It finally occurred to me that my symptoms were classic for posterior subcapsular cataracts. I had my partner examine my eyes and he confirmed the diagnosis. Since my story has become known, several prominent ophthalmologists have related similar sequences of known dry eyes confusing the diagnosis of cataracts.

I learned how poorly Snellen acuity reflects your real world vision. On the day of diagnosis, my vision was OD 20/20 and blurry with OS 20/25 and blurrier. I was dangerous driving at night. I could not drive toward the sun in the morning until about 10:00 am. Miraculously, I could operate through a microscope without difficulty and I could still perform oculoplastic surgery without loupes. I began to track my intraoperative complications leading up to my own surgery and afterward.

After being an eye surgeon for 10 years, I also learned how different glare and halos are to a patient. The Array surgeon needs to have a very clear understanding of these issues. Figure 17-2 shows a scene at dusk with a "normal" view. The image is not perfect. It has a visible glow, not a halo or glare, around several of the headlights. Figure 17-3 has halos or rings around the headlights. The rings in this picture are more pronounced than seen by most Array patients. Figure 17-4 has severe, poorly focused halos around the headlights. These rings are typical of the first few days after implantation with the Array. Figure 17-5 has starbursts on the headlights. Most Array patients do not see starbursts. This image is more typical of soft contact lens wearers. Figure 17-6 has minimal glare from cataracts around the headlights. Notice that the glare destroys the ability to see the front of the car while the halos allow you to visualize the front of the car. Figure 17-7 has significant glare from cataracts. The glare severely limits resolution within the entire picture. This is the amount of glare I had when my vision was 20/25 by Snellen acuity.

My IOL Decision

At this point, surgery was not an option; it was a matter of time. I had the opportunity to see the rapid deterioration of my vision from posterior subcapsular cataracts (PSC). When I had an image uniformly lit from the front, I could see very well. When an image had a strong source of light beside or behind it, I could barely see. I discovered the uniformly lit surgical field of an operating microscope always allowed me to see well. I could, however, track the growth of my PSCs by observing the slow, unrelenting growth of their shadows in the operating field. My worst problem was getting to and from work safely. I was fine once I arrived at work.

My partner, Michael G. Orr, MD, and I started implanting the Array multifocal IOL in March 1998. We tracked our outcomes very closely. We were impressed with how well our patients were seeing without glasses at distance and near. I became very interested in having the Array implanted in my eyes. Our concern was a lack of data. To our knowledge, no other ophthalmologist had been implanted with the Array IOL. I had a very helpful conversation with Ivan Marais, MD from South Africa who had implanted over 1000 of the Array Multifocal IOLs. He had implanted the lens in a gastroenterologist who had no difficulty seeing through an endoscope. According to this doctor, there were no halos seen when looking through the endoscope.

My motivation to try the Array was based on three pillars, the same three pillars I emphasize to my patients. I was extremely motivated to decrease my dependence on glasses, I was willing to put up with some visual aberrations to achieve my goal, and I knew I had a fantastic surgeon in my partner, who could take care of all of the usual cataract surgery issues and deal with my 1.5 D of preexisting corneal cylinder. We had been performing refractive cataract surgery on our patients for years. I needed bilateral implantation and was willing to step into the unknown to get what I wanted. I also knew Dr. Orr would exchange my Array IOLs if I complained enough.

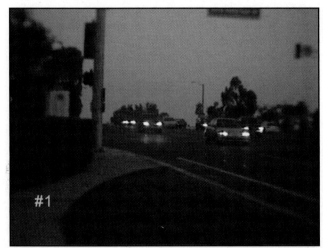

Figure 17-2. "Normal" view at dusk.

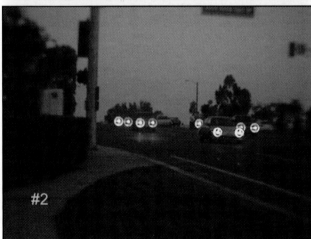

Figure 17-3. Halos around headlights.

My Surgical Experience

I had cataract surgery on my left eye on May 4, 1998 and my right eye on June 29, 1998. We separated the two eyes by 8 weeks to understand what the problems were with a cataract in one eye and an Array in the other eye. Dr. Orr performed both surgeries. He used intracameral anesthesia, approximately 1 cc of nonpreserved 1% lidocaine. He did superior limbal relaxing incisions. The capsulotomy was 5.5 mm in diameter and the Array multifocal IOL was injected into the capsular bag with the Unfolder.

I was amazed at my ability to see the surgery in progress. I could see the capsulotomy forceps tearing the anterior capsule and occasionally a glimmer from the torn capsular edge. I saw the fluid wave of the hydrodissection move across the lens. It created a dramatic opalescent effect within the lens. As soon as the fluid wave passed through the lens, it created thousands of diffracting points within the lens and the light show was absolutely amazing. The intense white light of the microscope was transformed into all of the colors of the rainbow, more vivid than I had ever seen. The light show diminished when the nucleus was removed, but lasted until the cortex was gone. I could see and hear the phacoemulsifier needle moving. During the irrigation and aspiration, I could see the cortex

Figure 17-4. Severe, poorly focused halos.

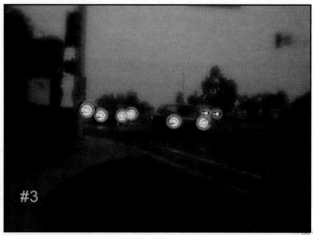

Figure 17-5. Starbursts on the headlight.

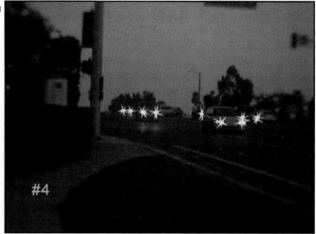

stripped toward the center of the capsule. I watched the lens unfold into the capsular bag without incident. I could follow the leading haptic into the bag. Once both haptics were in place, I could no longer see the IOL. I now use these experiences to talk my patients through their own surgical experience. The patient is uniformly comforted by my description of what they are about to see during their own intracameral anesthesia.

My postoperative course was similar between the two eyes. I was able to read a newspaper sitting in the recovery area several minutes after the surgery. I was able to see well at distance. The next day I was 20/15 and J_1 to J_1+ without correction. I was elated. The quality of my vision continued to get better for several days after each surgery. I had a waffle pattern of clear vision with vertical and horizontal blurred lines in my central vision for 2 days from intraoperative corneal bending. I could always see well through the waffle pattern, but having it disappear was very comforting.

My Experience Between Eyes

It was visually uncomfortable to have an Array multifocal IOL in my left eye and a posterior subcapsular cataract in my right eye. The two eyes had different optical systems and dissimilar images. My most important observation was that the dissimilar images

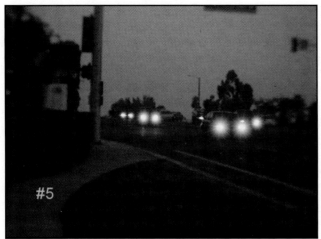

Figure 17-6. Minimal glare.

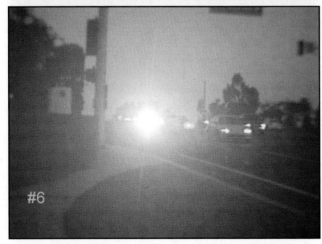

Figure 17-7. Significant glare.

were different at different distances. When I was driving, the continuously variable relationship of the images was very unsettling. Once I was able to understand their origin I could begin to ignore them. Once I was bilaterally implanted, the dissimilar images became similar and much less bothersome.

The two different images were most annoying because they were constantly changing relative to each other. The halos around lights with the Array IOL seemed to enlarge at certain distances. Many of my patients had reported that the halos were huge around headlights of a car. They seemed to be much bigger when the car was farther away from me. The glare of my PSC was minimal at a distance but grew progressively worse as the car approached. The halos were just the opposite. They grew smaller and smaller as the car approached. The difference was maddening and confusing.

It took me several weeks to understand the difference between my two eyes. The glare from the PSC was directly related to the intensity of the light source and inversely related to the darkness of the background. Therefore, the closer the headlight came toward me at night, the worse the glare became. The halos behaved differently at different distances. Inside of 100 feet, the halos got smaller as I got closer to them. They seemed to collapse onto the object creating them and disappear around 20 feet. Outside of 100 feet, the halos were relatively constant in size, but the objects around the halos were getting smaller. This gave the false impression that the halos were increasing in size. Once I realized that the objects were decreasing in size and that the halos were staying the same size, the difference between the two eyes bothered me less because it was more consistent with my prior experience. This is an important recurring theme in adaptation to the Array IOL. The patient needs to be able to understand the visual anomalies, to relate them to his or her prior visual experience and, ultimately, to ignore them.

After several weeks of using the Array IOL in one eye, I was ready to have my second eye implanted. I was ready because I had great vision in my eye with the Array IOL. I was ready because my vision was getting worse in my unoperated eye. Most of all, I was ready because I had already experienced the halos and dealt with them.

My Bilateral Array IOL Experience

My second eye was implanted with the Array IOL on June 29, 1998. I noticed the two eyes were working well together within a few minutes of the operation. I also noticed that the disparity between the two eyes was gone by the time I got to the recovery room. As soon as the second eye was implanted, the visual aberrations matched and became less noticeable to me. I still had the halos in both eyes; however, the halos and all of the other aberrations were similar between the two eyes, which made all of the difference to me.

Once I was bilaterally implanted with the Array IOL, I began to adapt to the unwanted visual images in a remarkable way. I had my second surgery on a Monday. I saw a full day of patients in the office on Wednesday and I operated all day Thursday and Friday. I was immediately able to use my new vision at home and at work. I could see perfectly through an operating microscope from the first week. I could read low-contrast material without difficulty, but I had to use reading glasses for high-contrast material such as a laser printed report. I could see well immediately; I had 20/15 uncorrected vision at distance, and J_1+ at near.

The most amazing aspect of my postoperative vision is that it got better with time. I gradually learned to ignore the parts of my vision that I did not want to see and I learned to enhance the images that I wanted to see. This adaptation continues today, 20 months after my second surgery, and I believe it will continue to improve for years to come. I compare it to how I must have learned to use my original visual system. It took me years to be able to reliably catch a baseball thrown to me. No doubt some of that learning was my visual system. I just know I learned to catch the ball, I didn't much care about the process. At 43 years old, I know the only parts of my body improving are my eyes and, if I wasn't an eye surgeon, I wouldn't much care about the process.

The Waltz Array Model

The Array IOL has a refractive, distance dominant, zonal progressive optic. There are five zones, and each zone has distance and near focusing capabilities in varying proportions. The central zone one is primarily for distance but has a small near effect. Zones two and four are primarily near. Zones three and five are weighted toward the distance. The net effect of the varying zones is highly pupil dependent. With a 2 mm pupil, the lens is similar to a monofocal IOL. As the pupil enlarges, the add power is unmasked and the near vision is enhanced. None of the incident light is lost to diffraction. Approximately 50% of the light is focused by the lens for distance, 13% for intermediate, and 37% for near, depending on the diameter of the pupil when the measurements are taken.

The Waltz Array model is a quick way to visualize how the Array IOL works in most situations. Imagine the Array IOL is 6 mm in diameter and has only two zones, a central 2 mm distance button and a doughnut shaped add that is 2 mm wide. We will ignore the intermediate portion for this simplification. The pupil size determines what part of the IOL "sees" incoming light and contributes to the retinal image.

When the pupil is constricted to 2 mm or less, the Array IOL is essentially a monofocal IOL. There is no secondary image or halos and there is no useful near vision. The patient will need bifocals to see well at near but will not have any unwanted visual images at distance or near. In bright light, my pupil is very small and I see extremely well at distance. My uncorrected vision is 20/10. I never see halos around lights, but I usually need reading glasses for near. When I use reading glasses in very bright light, my near vision is fantastic because I am moving my 20/10 distance vision to my near vision.

The annular bifocal is unmasked as the pupil dilates and two simultaneous images are created. By creating two images, I can avoid using reading glasses, but I always have an unwanted image to manage. The distance image is about one third brighter than the near image (50%/35%=1.35). This is a critical point because it explains the value of a slight loss in contrast sensitivity. When the patient is reading with the Array IOL's bifocal, the near image is in focus and the distance image is out-of-focus. The distance image is brighter and forms a halo around the letters. It is easier to ignore the unwanted images due to the slight loss in contrast sensitivity of the Array IOL, especially if there is less contrast between the printing and the paper. Less light on the page also makes the unwanted images easier to ignore.

By using this simple model of the Array IOL, you can accurately predict how to minimize the patient's unwanted visual images. For example, some patients will complain of a fuzzy image or halos at near but have great distance vision. Using our model, we know to suggest using a bright light to constrict the pupil and mask the annular near portion of the lens. Adding reading glasses will then bring the great distance vision to near and minimize the patient's complaints. You can reassure the patient that he or she will become less dependent on the reading glasses over time, typically several months.

We have reproduced a high contrast near card to illustrate the dual viewing options at near (Figure 17-8). The problems with the optics of the Array IOL have been exaggerated for this illustration. The left side of the near card is perfectly clear. I see this image when I use bright illumination to constrict my pupil and a +3.00 reading add. The right side of the near card is modified to simulate vision with the Array. There is a sharply focused image of each letter from the Array bifocal and an out-of-focus image of the same letter surrounding it from the central distance portion of the lens. You will notice the primary image is not blurred by the secondary image. There is also a very prominent packing effect with the secondary image. As the letters are placed closer together, the secondary images blend together. This decreases the contrast of the primary image and background, and helps the Array patient read letters that are relatively tightly packed better than widely spaced letters.

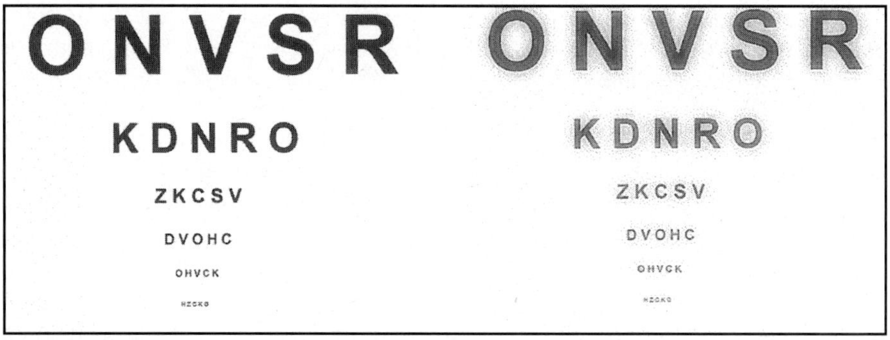

Figure 17-8. High contrast near card.

Images I See with the Array

The most important measure of how well the Array IOL has worked for me is my incidence of surgical complications. I tracked my surgical complications leading up to my own surgery and afterward. I had no intraoperative complications for the 6 months prior to becoming binocularly implanted with the Array, including the 8 weeks that I was monocularly implanted. I had no complications for the 4 months after being binocularly implanted. This strongly suggests that the Array works well in a microsurgical environment.

I see well with the Array IOL, but I do not see perfectly. I see halos around point sources of light at night. My intermediate vision is not great. I have a hard time reading high-contrast print in bright light. On the other hand, I read for hours in moderate to dim light without glasses. My vision is a 20/10 at distance without correction while I am wearing my sunglasses on the beach. I can operate with a microscope for hours without any visual fatigue. I never wear glasses while examining patients in the office because I can see everything I need to see without them.

My Recommendations for Patient Counseling

Patient selection begins with doctor selection. The Array surgeon must be a refractive cataract surgeon. Small incisions, astigmatic control, accurate IOL calculations, and rare complications need to be routine for the Array surgeon. If these issues are not given due consideration, the patient is less likely to be satisfied with his or her surgical outcome. The following discussion assumes state-of-the-art refractive cataract surgery.

The best indication for the Array IOL is a desire to be less dependent on glasses. Yet, one of the strongest contraindications is a demand to be completely independent of glasses or contacts. The ideal Array candidate has high visual demands, but realistic expectations, and is highly motivated to become less dependent on glasses. Although it is possible to be completely glasses free, it is unlikely and unwise to allow the patient to hope for such an outcome. There are no absolute contraindications to the Array IOL. The relative contraindications are fewer all of the time.

The best patient for the Array IOL is the low to moderate hyperope who is also presbyopic. These patients hate their glasses. They typically did not start wearing glasses until they were adults and did not incorporate glasses into their body image. Presbyopia was

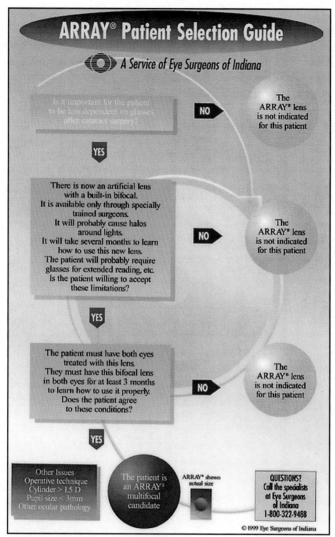

Figure 17-9. Array patient selection guide.

the gasoline thrown onto their smoldering discontent. They are uniformly excited about, and happy with, their Array IOL even when the refractive outcome is not ideal.

The most challenging Array patients are near emmetropic and not presbyopic. These patients already see well at distance and near and expect to see even better at distance and near postoperatively. I was emmetropic and not presbyopic preoperatively and I am very happy. The point is while anyone can benefit from the lens, some patients require more preoperative and postoperative counseling than others.

I screen all of my cataract patients preoperatively for suitability for the Array IOL. I ask them three questions to determine if they are likely to benefit from the Array. I use a form developed at my practice (Figure 17-9). If they answer all three questions positively, I will probably consider using the Array IOL.

I recommend the beginning Array surgeon start with low hyperopic presbyopes. This group is the most tolerant of imperfection with the Array IOL. Implant all of your early patients bilaterally. Implant five to 10 hyperopic presbyopic patients with the Array IOL, then stop implanting the Array IOL for 3 months. Talk to the patients when they return for follow-up. Learn what makes them happy. Learn what frustrates them with their vision. Implant another group and follow them for a while. You will discover a trend. No matter how well someone sees with the Array, he or she will see better several months later. Accept the fact that you will explant some lenses, because it will happen. Did you learn phaco without tearing a capsule? You will also learn that your happiest, most satisfied patients are patients with the Array IOL in both eyes.

REFERENCE

1. Javitt JC, Wang F, Trentacost DJ, et al. Outcomes of cataract extraction with multifocal intraocular lens implantation—Functional status and quality of life. *Ophthalmology*. 1997; 104:589-599.

18

Clear Lensectomy for Refractive Errors

Kurt A. Buzard, MD

INTRODUCTION

Among the oldest surgical procedures in ophthalmology are the various surgical treatments for cataracts. Beginning with primitive couching procedures used to force the lens out of the visual path, cataract surgery today has evolved into a highly refined and safe procedure with improvements not only in best-corrected vision, but in the number of patients who gain the ability to see well without glasses. The arrival of refractive phacoemulsification has significant implications for the cataract patient and for the field of refractive surgery in general. As is well known, there are two major refractive elements in the eye, and while the success of manipulation of the cornea for refractive surgery is well known, lens-based surgical manipulation may well be the hallmark of the next era of refractive surgery, either with or without the removal of the natural crystalline lens.

Since the IOL has been available and in widespread use for many years, why has it taken until now to embrace the concept of refractive manipulation of the lens? The answer, to put it in a nutshell, is technology and technique. Even though the IOL—and before it phacoemulsification—were available, reliable positioning and non-invasive placement were problematic. Prior to the capsulorrhexis technique, reliable placement of the IOL in the bag was hit and miss, leading to variation of the resulting refraction. In addition, accurate measurement of axial length and corneal curvature, and/or calculation of IOL power were subject to unacceptable inaccuracies. With the larger wounds required by rigid PMMA IOLs, ocular integrity and intraocular pressure were often compromised, leading to disruption of intraocular contents and higher rates of retinal detachment and infection. In addition, the larger wounds led to iatrogenic astigmatism, which often progressed over time. Again, correction of astigmatism was possible using corneal incisions but required a trip to the operating room or equivalent, with the expense and time costs became prohibitive for the majority of patients. Additionally, measurement of the appropriate IOL power has only gradually improved to the point that reliable refractive results can be expected. Any refractive operation must have safe and reliable enhancements. The development of 3.0 mm IOL exchange through the original incision has allowed a lens-based enhancement to become a reality. The answer to the question of why it has taken until now to develop true refractive phacoemulsification is a sum of many small and large advances, which taken together have led to a revolution in lens-based refractive surgery.

While improvements in the treatment of myopia and astigmatism in virtually all degrees have been frequent and ongoing, the treatment of hyperopia has noticeably lagged. Many operations have been proposed and investigated with equivocal or poor results. Much of the problem resides in the attempt to create hyperopic corrections within the cornea, which seems to have been less successful than corresponding myopic corrections. Initially, the most common form of hyperopia was iatrogenic, aphakia-induced by cataract extraction without the implantation of an IOL. Attempts to correct aphakia with keratophakia, epikeratophakia, and intracorneal lenses resulted in intermittent acceptable results with many complications, including irregular astigmatism. For correction of both extreme myopia and hyperopia, limitations exist with respect to maximum and minimum corneal curvatures. It is generally accepted that the initial statement made by Dr. José Barraquer that the maximum corneal curvature should be less than 50 and greater than 35 seems to hold true today. Additionally, limitations exist with respect to the minimum residual corneal thickness in the bed of lamellar refractive procedures, which is felt to be a minimum of 250 microns. While the introduction of the IOL effectively resolved the issue of aphakia, gradual improvements in the surgical incision, phacoemulsification, and calculation of the lens power have resulted in an operation with improved accuracy and safety to warrant the refractive designation.

This chapter will support the thesis that the majority of patients over age 50 with hyperopia and extreme myopia, are best treated by exchange of the crystalline lens rather than an operation involving the cornea. In fact, I prefer to call this procedure lens exchange rather than clear lens extraction since we believe the latter name is pejorative (many, if not most, of the patients in their 50s have incipient lens changes), while the former name speaks to the refractive changes intended by the operation (exchange of a lens incapable of producing good uncorrected vision for one that is capable of emmetropia). It is my contention that for patients over the age of 50, the lens is a vestigial organ (much like the appendix) and for reasons of improved results, stabilization of the refraction, and the removal of any future cataract lens-based surgery is preferred. Hyperopic correction with lens surgery in excess of 2 to 3 D results in an operation with less glare, fewer complications, and better vision than corresponding corneal refractive options.

INCIDENCE AND CLASSIFICATION OF HYPEROPIA

Most studies of refractive error in infants have concluded that newborns are hyperopic with a broad distribution of refractive errors.[1] Within the first few years of life, the eye grows and most children shift toward emmetropia resulting in a steady decrease in the prevalence of hyperopia.[2] The hyperopia that remains results in an eye that is distinctly different from a normal or myopic eye because of its shorter axial length, shallower anterior chamber depth, and a flatter cornea.[3] These hyperopic patients often have strabismus problems and fight amblyopia during their childhood. As a result, many patients with congenital hyperopia have best-corrected vision of less than 20/20 in one or both eyes.

A distinctly different second group of hyperopes appears over age 50 with the hyperopic shift associated with aging. These patients often have a refraction that changes with time and the effects of aging on the lens. These patients have relatively low degrees of hyperopia in the range of 1 to 2 D and suffer from both hyperopia and presbyopia. The classification and treatment of hyperopia should therefore reflect the basic epidemiology of hyperopic patients. I therefore define low hyperopia as 0 to 2 D, moderate hyperopia from 2 to 6 D, and high hyperopia above 6 D. In addition, we qualify the use of lens exchange on two basic principles: age over 50 and/or hyperopia greater than 2 D, above which we believe the results of corneal hyperopic refractive surgery are less satisfactory at this time. Hyperopia is relatively uncommon until the age of 50, at which time there is a marked increase in hyperopia. The incidence of hyperopia is much more common at age 65 to 74 (67%) than it is at 43 to 54 (22%).[4]

The purpose of this chapter is to propose clear lens extraction with IOL implantation as the primary means of correcting hyperopia, high myopia, and in all patients other than those with accommodation (and even in patients with accommodation), if hyperopia is greater than 2 to 3 D. Previous articles have demonstrated both the good results associated with clear lens extraction[5,6] with small numbers and the relatively poor results obtained with hexagonal keratotomy,[7-13] epikeratophakia,[14-18] hyperopic ALK,[19] thermokeratoplasty,[20-23] and even hyperopic PRK and LASIK.[24-26] While hyperopic PRK and LASIK have promise for producing better results than the others, particularly with adjustments to the ablation profile, it remains true that most of these patients are in their mid to late 50s with at least mild lens changes, which, in my opinion, substantially alters the appropriate mode of action. Even if corneal operations were markedly successful for hyperopia, subsequent lens changes will lead to changes in refractive errors. Even the application of photorefractive keratectomy may well promote the onset of these lens changes. These important issues have not been properly addressed in previous studies when considering the correction of hyperopia. In the instance of a patient 30 to 40 years old with myopia or mild hyperopia, a reasonable expectation of 10 to 20 years of benefit can be expected. Whereas in a patient in his or her late 50s with early lens changes, a corneal operation is unlikely to provide benefit for more than 5 to 10 years. In distinction, a clear lens extraction with IOL implantation can provide a correction with the same duration as the myopic operation, at least 10 to 20 years. All of this points to the need to consider the patient over age 50 in a separate category and to place lens extraction as a primary modality.

RISK

Every surgical procedure has risk, and lens exchange is no exception. The primary areas of risk are retinal detachment, endophthalmitis, expulsive hemorrhage, vitreous loss/torn capsule/retained nuclear fragments, endothelial damage, and/or wound incompetence. Using the transconjunctival "blue line" incision, wound incompetence is virtually unknown. In approximately 5000 cases using this incision we have never had a wound leak, and historically the scleral tunnel incision has been shown to be a remarkably stable and strong incision, particularly if it is kept within the "incisional funnel."[27,28] Endophthalmitis has been reported as a problem with the clear corneal incision.[29] The wound construction can be relatively easily compromised, resulting in wound leakage and a setup for endophthalmitis. This is a strong incentive to consider the blue line incision in addition to the relative astigmatic neutrality of this wound construction. Any intraocular surgery is associated with some endothelial cell loss and, of course, IOLs placed in the anterior chamber are more likely to encounter this problem.[30,31] Werblin studied the issue of long-term endothelial stability after IOL implantation in several models using different types of IOLs.[32] He found that posterior chamber IOL implantation after phacoemulsification was associated with about a 10% cell loss that was stable after 3 years in patients followed up to 6 years. Problems with rupture of the capsule and/or vitreous loss should be rare in the relatively young patients with soft nuclei, but it is important to note that technique-related issues should be resolved before entering into lens exchange surgery. With good technique, related problems such as cystoid macular edema (CME) should be rare.[33] Similarly, with larger incisions that were not self-sealing and with older patients, expulsive hemorrhage was a more significant complication. This complication is rare in younger patients. With a small, self-sealing incision, it should be easy to raise IOP and inhibit progression of this problem.

The area of greatest concern is the problem of retinal detachment associated with lens extraction. At greater risk are those patients with myopia since retinal detachment rates are much lower for patients with hyperopia, and the results of lens exchange have been relatively good.[34-36] Few results are available for clear lens exchange in myopia, so most studies examine the rates of retinal detachment in cataract patients. By their nature, these patients are usually older with more difficult surgery; therefore; the rates should only be taken as a general measure of the actual rate. The most common studies involve older surgical techniques, yielding retinal detachment larger wounds and without capsulorrhexis with rates of 1.3 to 6% per year for ECCE surgeries.[37,38] In patients with high myopia (>10 D), the natural rate of retinal detachment is approximately 0.7% per year,[39] so the rate of retinal detachment is increased with ECCE surgeries and particularly after YAG laser capsulotomy. These studies point to the importance of maintaining the lens-iris diaphragm to minimize the movement of vitreous, and without an intact posterior capsule, the barrier is incomplete. We create an anterior capsulotomy smaller than the IOL optic (usually about 5 mm), and when YAG laser is performed, the opening is made through an undilated pupil (approximately 4 mm). This ensures a tight lens-iris diaphragm and minimal movement of vitreous. Verzella performed one of the earliest and largest studies of lens exchange in high myopia and reported a retinal detachment rate of only 0.7%,[40,41] approximately the same as the rate without lens surgery. Unfortunately, the visual results were less than impressive, with 89% within 6 D of the intended correction due in large part to a limited range of available IOL powers. While Verzella required preoperative and yearly retinal checks, other authors have insisted on prophylactic retinal treatments, apparently with relatively good results.

Colin[42] studied 49 eyes of 28 patients with approximately two-thirds treated with retinal photocoagulation prior to surgery. With a 4-year follow-up, the incidence of retinal detachment was 1.9% and the incidence of YAG capsulotomy was 36.7%. Uncorrected visual acuity of 20/40 or better was achieved in 38% of patients. Eighty-two percent treated with YAG laser had 20/100 or better versus 62% of untreated eyes. The increased rate of retinal detachment, which he has recently reported to be even higher, might be explained by the fact that some of the patients underwent ECCE. Failure of prophylactic photocoagulation might also have been a factor.

Centurion[44] has reported on high myopes who were treated preoperatively with prophylactic photocoagulation and followed for 6 years. In 35 patients, no retinal detachments were noted after cataract surgery, although the visual results were again a little disappointing with only 75% of the patients with 2 D or less of residual myopia.

SURGICAL TECHNIQUE

The surgical technique is essentially the same as cataract surgery, but some important points need to be made. Much of the discussion with lens exchange has resolved around complications. However, the actual technique is also important, not only with regard to the initial procedure, but with regard to "enhancement procedures" as well. We believe that it is important to maintain ocular pressure during the procedure and that failure to do so may result in higher rates of retinal detachment. Additionally, as discussed above, we use a 5 mm capsulorrhexis and a small YAG laser capsulotomy when required. Clearly, any complication is magnified with a surgical procedure that is cosmetic. With this in mind, the surgeon should carefully evaluate each aspect of the procedure, particularly as it relates to complications, especially infection. This is particularly true as it relates to the choice of incision. While the clear corneal incision can be performed without complication in the majority of patients, it is relatively unforgiving and more likely to leak. A clear corneal incision may allow for a higher incidence of infection than a scleral tunnel incision.

The surgeon should review his or her results with respect to refractive outcomes. If uncorrected vision is not better than 20/40 in the majority of patients, a possible review of both preoperative workup and surgical technique may be appropriate before making the move to refractive lens exchange. Additionally, any refractive procedure requires the ability to enhance the result, and the surgeon should consider whether his or her ability to enhance both astigmatic and spherical results after the original surgery are adequate and, equally important, cost-effective. LASIK may be used to correct both astigmatic and spherical errors, but in most cases will not be a cost-effective procedure unless utilized in small numbers. Additionally, LASIK in the older patient, in our experience, is often complicated by epithelial disruption that can result in prolonged visual recovery. I will describe three basic techniques that form the basics of "lens exchange" in my practice: the basic lens removal technique, the 3 mm sutureless IOL exchange technique, and the technique for slit lamp astigmatic keratotomy.

Basic Lens Removal Technique

There are as many ways to remove a lens as there are surgeons, but in very general terms we use the blue line cataract incision (a transconjunctival incision created with a diamond blade), and we do not believe in the use of limbal relaxing incisions at the time of cataract surgery because of their limited effect and possible long-term instability. This technique is described in more detail in a recent publication.

I usually perform the blue line incision superiorly, although it may be applied in any meridian. I utilize a trapezoid diamond knife (Buzard Blue Line knife from Mastel Precision). The diamond has a 2.7 mm inside width, a 3.0 mm outside width, and is 6 mm long with a truncated tip 100 microns in length to provide better control during creation of the incision. Of particular interest, the blade of the knife is at least 2 mm longer than the standard cataract diamond knife, allowing for the more posterior placement of the external wound and generally a longer tunnel incision.

The eye is stabilized by grasping in the inferior conjunctiva and drawing the eye downward with a .5 forceps. The blue line incision is constructed by first creating, with the side of the diamond knife, a 4.00 mm incision through the conjunctiva about 1.5 to 2.0 mm behind the surgical limbus (represented by an anatomic appearance of a blue line)

(Figures 18-1a and 18-1b). In the usual case, the conjunctiva will sag naturally away from the incision and the resulting conjunctival gaping will create a "mini-peritomy"(Figure 18-2a). While bleeding is not a significant problem, the assistant applies steady drops to maintain visualization of the exterior incision. The knife is placed parallel to the posterior sclera, and pressure is applied to slightly indent the sclera, with the knife pushing forward to begin the scleral tunnel incision (Figure 18-2b). As the incision evolves, progressive pressure is placed on the heel of the diamond knife to prevent early interior entry caused by the changing curvature at the limbus between sclera and cornea (Figure 18-2c). Finally, when the tip of the knife approaches the desired location for the internal corneal incision, the heel of the knife is rotated slightly upward, creating a slight dimple in the corneal surface. The corneal dimple is relieved when the tip of the knife penetrates Descemet's membrane (Figure 18-2d). The knife is then inserted until the "shoulders" are at the level of the internal corneal incision, which is 2.7 mm in width. The blue line incision described above results in an approximately 3 x 3 mm square scleral tunnel incision. Light cautery is then applied to the conjunctival edge to control bleeding. A side-port incision is made with the same diamond knife, viscoelastic is instilled in the anterior chamber, and the capsulorrhexis is performed with a cystotome. Hydrodissection and hydrodelineation are performed, and a derivation of the standard divide and conquer phacoemulsification technique is used to remove the soft lens. At present, I like the Staar three-piece silicone IOL with a 6.30 optic and a 13.50 overall length (Staar Surgical Company, Monravia, Calif). I like this lens because it goes in through a very small incision and is easy to remove during IOL exchange, which I will discuss next. Viscoelastic material is removed with irrigation and aspiration. A wound leakage test is performed by injecting saline through the side-port, then checking along the incision and on the sclera. The appearance of the final wound is shown in Figure 18-3. Of interest is the fact that hydration of the cornea, frequently required to obtain a watertight wound in the clear corneal incision (about 20% in our hands), is rarely required with the blue line incision (about 5%).

3 mm IOL Exchange

The ability to safely and reliably exchange the IOL is a key to the refractive designation of the procedure. In addition, I prefer to use the original incision so as to minimize iatrogenic trauma to the eye. To reopen the incision, I use the tip of the diamond knife to trace the external opening of the original incision and to begin a dissection in the scleral bed. At this point, if the proper plane has been identified, a cyclodialysis spatula may be used to reopen the original incision. I have been able to reopen incisions up to 6 months after the original surgery with little effort. If the incision does not open easily, the truncated tip of the diamond knife will usually follow the same path and can be used as a sharp dissection tool to reopen the incision. I create the side-port incision as a beveled incision and make the same attempt to reopen this incision with the same knife. Some surgeons have been concerned that reopening the original incision may lead to difficulties in closure or healing, but it has been my experience that these difficulties do not usually occur. In most cases, the incision closes without sutures. Occasionally, a horizontal suture may be used for closure, particularly if vitreous has been encountered, but in most cases it is unnecessary.

One advantage of the silicone Staar three-piece IOL is that it does not stick to the capsule, and if the original surgery was atraumatic to the bag and/or zonular attachments,

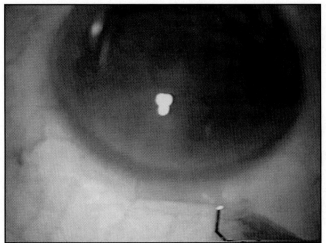

Figure 18-1a. Anatomy and positioning of the transconjunctival blue line incision.

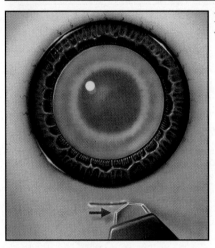

Figure 18-1b. Illustration of the transconjunctival blue line incision.

the IOL may be dislodged relatively easily in the first 3 months and even up to a year if the conditions are right. One thing that helps in this regard is a clean and well-polished bag, which is then less likely to stick firmly together. I have found that it is generally unwise to exchange the IOL after YAG laser capsulotomy since the capsule almost invariably tears. An alternative strategy for this situation is to add a low diopter IOL (available from Staar from -6 to +6 in 1 D increments) in the sulcus as a piggyback lens. This approach is acceptable in the circumstance of a previous YAG laser capsulotomy, but we feel that a lens exchange is preferable since only one lens will be present and standard IOLs are available in 0.5 D increments.

After reopening the incision, I inject viscoelastic into the anterior chamber and dislodge the IOL with a side movement and injection of viscoelastic into the bag. I then utilize a Bond straight hook to engage the inferior haptic and rotate it out of the bag. The same hook can be used to move the opposing haptic from the bag and present the IOL in the anterior chamber. The superior haptic is then engaged and drawn through the incision. Viscoelastic is used to push the IOL away from the cornea; the lens is now in position to be bisected with a stainless steel snare. The snare (Geuder product #G-32800) is

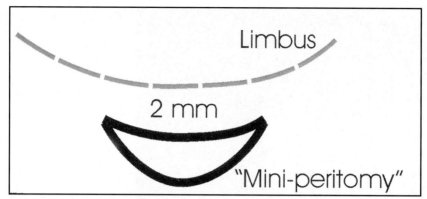

Figure 18-2a. Illustration of positioning of the blue line incision with automatic creation of a "mini-peritomy."

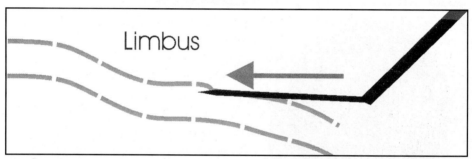

Figure 18-2b. Illustration of the creation of the incision by first pressing flat against the conjunctiva.

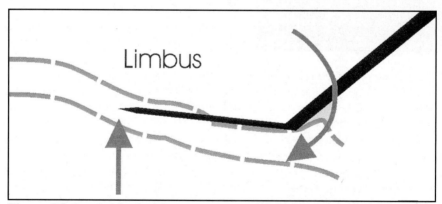

Figure 18-2c. As the incision progresses, the heel of the blade is pressed downward to rotate the tip of the knife upwards as the tip enters clear cornea.

prepared, with bending, to enlarge the opening. Failure to enlarge the opening will result in snagging of the snare on the lens and difficulty in proper positioning. The snare is then placed around the exterior haptic and midway on the optic within the eye. The instrument is then used to bisect the IOL (Figure 18-4). The halves are removed with a 0.12

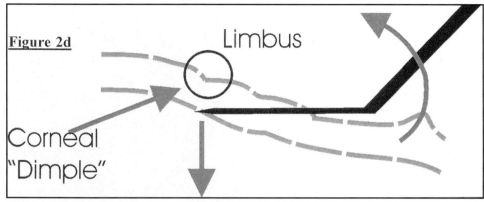

Figure 18-2d. When the appropriate length of incision has been reached the heel of the blade is rotated upwards, creating a "dimple" on the corneal surface.

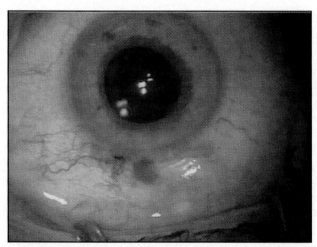

Figure 18-3. The appearance of the incision at the conclusion of surgery showing absence of chemosis, position of the incision, "automatic peritomy," and watertight closure.

toothed forceps. The eye is then ready to accept the replacement IOL, which is inserted in the usual manner.

My results with this technique have been excellent, with no significant complications. I calculate the power of the replacement lens based on the postoperative refraction rather than the axial length and test the patient with a soft contact lens prior to replacement.

Slit Lamp Astigmatic Correction

In true refractive surgery, correction of emmetropia must be exact and not an approximation of the actual problem or the final uncorrected vision will suffer. My assessment of limbal relaxing incisions is that the procedure fails to accurately correct pre-existing astigmatism and does not address the issue of induced astigmatism at all. Arcuate relaxing incisions have been proven over time to correct astigmatism in an accurate manner.[46] The problem with classic relaxing incisions is that they traditionally have been performed in an operating room (OR) or at least a minor surgery setting, increasing the time and cost

Figure 18-4. Illustration of the Geuder IOL snare in use to bisect the silicone IOL.

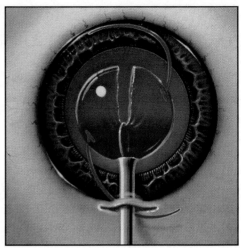

to the surgeon and patient. For over 15 years I have performed incisional keratotomy at the slit lamp,[47] and the results have been both safe and effective. The advantages of surgery at the slit lamp are many, but primarily they allow the surgeon to apply the astigmatic correction at the time in the postoperative course that is appropriate and convenient for both surgeon and patient, with less concern for time and cost. In this vein, the relaxing incisions may be enhanced on demand, and the need for exact correction is lessened, leading to decreased overcorrection and complications related to the surgical technique.

The technique is relatively simple but needs to be practiced at the slit lamp prior to actual surgery. One good method of practice is a special device that holds an eyebank or pig eye in position to practice the technique. This device is available from Eduardo Arenas (Trans. 21 No. 100-20 70. Piso, Bogata, Colombia) and should be used prior to clinical implementation of the technique.

This technique is simply an adaptation of the technique used in the OR. We use a 7 mm optical zone (OZ) that is marked with a gentian violet marking pen and used to mark the OZ centered on the pupil. We use an Osher diamond knife with the head tilted at 45% to allow good visualization of the knife blade at the slit lamp (Figure 18-5). The diamond knife is set at 0.5 mm without regard to pachymetry and arcuate incisions are created according to a published nomogram.[47] A slight undercorrection is always advisable since retreatment is just as simple as the original procedure. The difference between slit lamp surgery and surgery in the OR is mainly in the way the surgeon's hand and the patient's eye are stabilized, and in the movement of the knife. In the OR, the hand is stabilized at the wrist and only the hand moves. At the slit lamp, the arm is stabilized by the elbow on the table and the wrist at the headrest (Figures 18-6a and 18-6b). In this case, the patient is asked to move his or her eye to make the appropriate incisions. Tobradex is prescribed for 4 to 7 days and the visual improvement is usually immediate.

SMALL CLINICAL STUDY

I performed clear lens exchange on 68 eyes of 34 patients ranging in age from 30 to 67 years old (average 52 ± 9 years) (Figure 18-7). Of these, 13 of the patients were male

Figure 18-5. Slit lamp appearance of diamond blade and footplates showing excellent visualization with angled knife design.

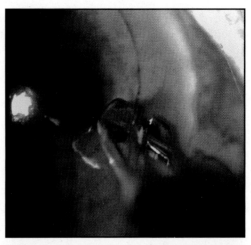

Figure 18-6a. Illustration of positioning of elbow against table and wrist against chinrest on the slit lamp to stabilize the arm during slit lamp astigmatic surgery.

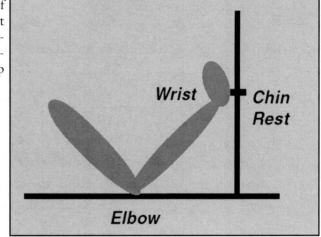

and 21 were female. Of these eyes, 25 were performed for a monovision correction, while 43 were corrected for distance. Surgery was performed on an outpatient basis using either a sutureless incision (57 eyes) or a single horizontal suture (11 eyes) in patients in whom a foldable lens could not be obtained to meet the power requirements for their eye.

Mean best-corrected vision prior to surgery was 20/20, while mean preoperative uncorrected vision was 20/100. Mean preoperative spherical equivalent for hyperopic patients was +2.72 + 1.59 D (Figure 18-8), while mean spherical equivalent for the myopic patients was -12.30 + 7.94 D. Mean keratometry was 43.65 + 2.13 and average cell count was 2700 cells\mm^2 prior to surgery.

Preoperatively, the same general routine used for our cataract patients was followed. All eyes were examined for systemic problems. Ocular examination included corrected and uncorrected distance visual acuity, manifest refraction, keratometry (Humphrey), corneal topography (EyeSys), cell count (Konan), and axial length (Nidek). Calculations were done using the Hoffer IOL calculation computer program aiming for a postoperative spherical equivalent value of -0.50 D for distance, and reading values using a "mono-

Figure 18-6b. At the slit lamp, the arm is stabilized by the elbow on the table and the wrist at the head rest.

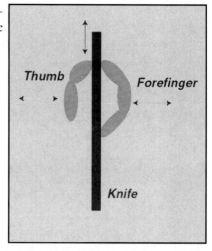

Figure 18-7. Preoperative distribution of age for all patients and for hyperopic patients.

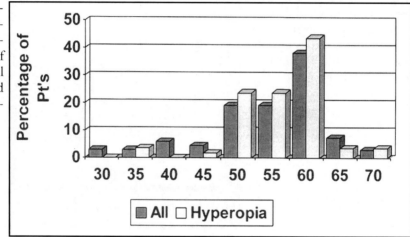

vision" system dependent on patient desires and testing prior to surgery, usually aiming for a postoperative result of -1.50 to –2.00 D in the reading eye.

RESULTS

No significant operative or postoperative complications were seen. Notably, no retinal complications occurred. The average postoperative spherical equivalent was -0.11 + 0.43 D for the distance eyes (Figure 18-9) and -1.79 + 0.53 D for the monovision eyes (Figure 18-10). The near correction results corresponded closely to the intended goal of -1.5 to -1.75 D correction of monovision in the reading eye. All refractions seemed relatively stable after that point. The mean uncorrected visual acuity improved from 20/100 preoperatively to an average of 20/30 with no lines lost on best-corrected visual acuity (BCVA) (Figure 18-11). The figure of 20/30 uncorrected vision included some patients in whom best-corrected vision was less than 20/20 due to refractive amblyopia. The average percentage of endothelial cell loss measured at the 6-month visit was 9.8 + 2.1%. Average preoperative astigmatism was 0.94 D (range 2.88 D to 0.25 D) for patients with

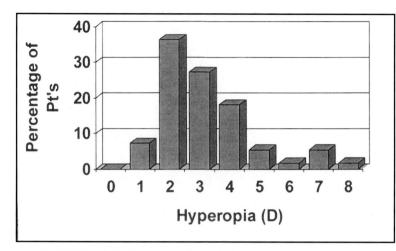

Figure 18-8. Preoperative distribution of spherical equivalent for hyperopic patients.

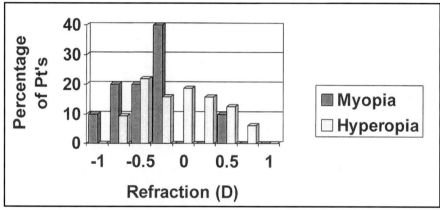

Figure 18-9. Postoperative distribution of spherical equivalent for myopic and hyperopic patients showing all patients in the study ± 1 D.

near corrections and 1.27 D (range 4.38 D to 0.00 D) for patients for distance correction. Astigmatic relaxing incisions were performed in 25 eyes with reduction of postoperative astigmatism to under 1 D in all patients. All patients seemed satisfied with the surgery. In particular, the patients were happy with the monovision corrections, which were heavily dependent on careful preoperative discussion and assessment of success with monovision by means of contact lens trials and teaching.

Enhancement operations were necessary in a total of 17 patients, in addition to the aforementioned 25 patients treated at the slit lamp with relaxing incisions for astigmatism. One patient was treated with LASIK for mild unexpected myopia and one patient was treated with LASIK to reverse a monovision correction. A 3 mm, sutureless IOL exchange was necessary in three patients due to residual hyperopia. No complications were encountered with any of these enhancements.

Figure 18-10. Postoperative distribution of spherical equivalent for reading eyes of monovision patients.

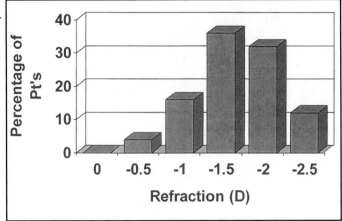

Figure 18-11. Postoperative distribution of uncorrected visual acuity.

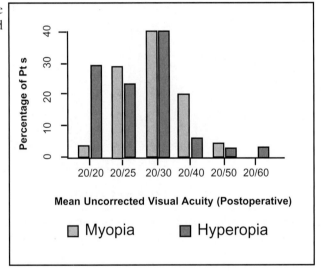

DISCUSSION

The concept of clear lens extraction with IOL implantation is not new and has been proposed previously by other authors.[44,45] What have not changed are the relatively poor results obtained with corneal manipulation for hyperopia, even with newer techniques of thermokeratoplasty, hyperopic PRK, and hyperopic LASIK. For small amounts of hyperopic correction (under 2 to 4 D), these corneal techniques can be successful with minimal loss of best-corrected visual acuity and few complications. However, for larger degrees of hyperopia, there seems to be a common problem experienced by virtually all corneal hyperopic procedures, which is loss of best-corrected visual acuity with even very mild decentrations of the procedure. Why the cornea tolerates relatively large decentrations for myopic procedures, and not hyperopic or steepening procedures, is somewhat of a mystery. In addition, man, if not most of the patients presenting for hyperopic corrections are in the age group of 50 and older. In fact, most are in their mid to late 50s. As patients enter in to the middle and late 50s, lens changes begin to occur that cannot be classified as cataracts, but under conditions of bright or poor lighting, these can result in a loss of detail, which may be noticeable to the patient following a corneal refractive procedure. We have observed several patients with such lens changes that underwent myopic or hyperopic LASIK procedures with resulting best-corrected vision of 20/25 to 20/30 and significant complaints of poor vision with increased glare following the procedure. Observation at the slit lamp revealed small increases in nuclear sclerosis and often the development of subtle anterior and posterior subcapsular changes. Removal of the lenses and substitution with IOLs resolved the complaints in all of these patients and resulted in best-corrected vision of 20/20 in most of these cases. For this reason, and because even mild lenticular changes can result in refractive changes that can alter the refractive effect of corneal surgery, I now carefully evaluate even mild lenticular changes in patients 50 years and older for both myopic and hyperopic surgeries. If sufficient changes are present, as evidenced by slit lamp observation and/or glare, lens surgery is chosen to correct the refractive error rather than laser corneal surgery. In fact, lens refractive surgery has become the surgery of choice for patients older than age 50, and the use of LASIK in these patients is for special cases rather than the surgery of choice.

As a final inducement to consider lens replacement as a preferred treatment for hyperopia, and in general for patients over age 50, we note the markedly improved surgical techniques now available for cataract surgery. The small incision lens extraction with capsulorrhexis is much safer due to the self-sealing nature of the incision and maintenance of the anterior chamber during even violent patient movement and/or coughing. In the bag placement with the capsulorrhexis provides a superior fixation of the IOLs with subsequent improvement of refractive results, which have already been improved by better calculation formulas prior to surgery. In fact, the utilization of lens replacement surgery is really a reflection of our changing attitudes toward cataract surgery as a whole. Today, it is our goal to provide every cataract patient with an uncorrected postoperative visual acuity of 20/40 or better, and we reach this goal in our general population of cataract patients in more than 90% of the cases, often on the first day after surgery. This attitude is not unique to us, but in fact has become a common goal in many, if not most, of the cataract practices in the United States. If the "value added" refractive results, which can be obtained with small-incision sutureless cataract surgery and relatively minor astigmatic corrections, are made available to patients with cataracts, why then should they be denied to younger patients? The only subset of patients who might give a second thought to lens corrective surgery would be patients with active accommodation below the age of 38 to 40. However, in our experience, patients with severe degrees of hyperopia (greater than 2 to 3 D) are more than willing to give up accommodation for better uncorrected vision, as evidenced by a 32-year-old patient included in our study with 6 D of hyperopia preoperatively and 20/25 to 20/30 vision postoperatively. This patient is absolutely thrilled with the results of his surgery and feels the loss of accommodation was a minor price to pay for the resolution of his hyperopia. While all younger patients may not have the same response, it is certainly present in some patients. For those who desire an alternative, this relatively small group of patients might benefit from the ICL (intraocular phakic contact lens). Myopic patients have the additional consideration of possible retinal detachment, but this complication seems markedly decreased with more recent techniques and may even be reduced if appropriate retinal consultation is obtained. Even if retinal detachment occurs, modern retinal reattachment can be very successful; if the retinal detachment occurs years after the surgery, it is not entirely clear that the detachment is related to the lens exchange surgery.

In summary, clear lens extraction is a safe and predictable means to correct refractive errors of virtually any degree. The recent advances in wound construction and cataract removal have made clear lens extraction a natural outgrowth of the trend toward refractive phacoemulsification occurring in cataract surgery as a whole. Finally, the issue of early lenticular changes in patients over age 50 with the possibility of progression of these lenticular deficits with the application of the excimer laser makes clear lens extraction a superior approach for this particular group.

REFERENCES

1. Bullimore MA, Gilmartin B. *Surgery for Hyperopia and Presbyopia*. Baltimore, Md: Williams and Wilkins;1987.

2. van Alphern, GWHM. O emmetropia and ametropia. *Ophthalmologica Supplementum*. 1961;142(supp):1-92.

3. Sorsby A, Benjamin B, Davey, JB et al. *Emmetropia and its Aberrations*. London: Her Majesty's Stationery Office No. 293. 1957.

4. Wang Q, Klein BEK, Klein R, et al. Refractive status in the Beaver Dam eye study. *Invest Ophthalmol Vis Sci*. 1994;35:4344-4347.

5. Isfahani AH, Salz J. *Surgery for Hyperopia and Presbyopia*. Baltimore, Md: Williams & Wilkins; 1987.

6. Buzard KA, Fundingsland BR. *Clear Lens Extraction for Hyperopia Operative Techniques in Cataract and Refractive Surgery*. 1999;2:35-40.

7. Werblin TP. Hexagonal keratotomy-should we still be trying? *J Cataract Refract Surg*. 1996;12:613-620.

8. Grandon SC, Sanders DR, Anello RD, et al. Clinical evaluation of hexagonal keratotomy for the treatment of primary hyperopia. *J Cataract Refract Surg*. 1995;21:140-149.

9. Grady FJ. Hexagonal keratotomy for corneal steepening. *Ophthalmic Surg*. 1988;19:622-623.

10. Basuk WL, Zisman M, Waring GO, et al. Complications of hexagonal keratotomy. *Am J Ophthalmol*. 1994;117:37-49.

11. Mendez A. Hexagonal keratotomy for hyperopia. Paper presented at: The proceedings of the Keratorefractive Society; 1986; New Orleans, La.

12. Jensen RP. Hexagonal keratotomy: clinical experience with 483 eyes. *Int Ophthalmol Clin*. 1991;31:69-73.

13. Neumann AC, McCarty GR. Hexagonal keratotomy for correction of low hyperopia: preliminary results of a prospective study. *J Cataract Refract Surg*. 1988;14:265-269.

14. American Academy of Ophthalmology. Ophthalmic procedures assessment, keratophakia and keratomileusis: safety and effectiveness. *Ophthalmology*. 1992;99(8):1332-1341.

15. Ehrlich MI, Nordan LT. Epikeratophakia for the treatment of hyperopia. *J Cataract Refract Surg*. 1989;15:661-666.

16. McDonald MB, Kaufman HE, Aquavella JV, et al. The nationwide study of epikeratophakia for aphakia in adults. *Am J Ophthalmol*. 1987;103:358-365.

17. Arffa RC, Marelli TL, Morgan KS. Long-term follow-up refractive and keratometric results of pediatric epikeratophakia. *Arch Ophthmol*. 1986;104:668-670.

18. Dingeldein SA, McDonald MB. Epikeratophakia. *Int Ophthamol Clin*. 1988;28:134-144.

19. Manche EE, Judge A, Maloney RK. Lamellar keratoplasty for hyperopia. *J Refract Surg*. 1996;12:42-49.

20. Neumann AC, Fyodorov S, Sander DR. Radial thermokeratoplasty for the correction of hyperopia. *Refract Corneal Surg*. 1990;6:404-412.

21. Fyodorov SN, Ivashina AI, Aleksandrova OG, et al. Surgical correction of compound hypermetropic and mixed astigmatism by sectoral thermal keratocoagulation. *Implants in Ophthalmology*. 1990;2:43-48.

22. Neumann AC, Sanders D, Raanan M, et al. Hyperopic thermokeratoplasty: clinical evaluation. *J Cataract Refract Surg*. 1991;17:830-838.

23. Feldman ST, Ellis W, Frucht-Pery J, et al. Regression of effect following radial thermokeratoplasty in humans. *Refract Corneal Surg*. 1989;5:288-291.

24. Dausch D, Klein R, Schroder E. Excimer laser photorefractive keratectomy for hyperopia. *J Refract Corneal Surg*. 1993;9:20-28.

25. Dausch D, Klein R, Landesz M, Schroder E. Photorefractive keratectomy to correct astigmatism with myopia of hyperopia. *J Cataract Refract Surg*. 1994;20(suppl):252-257.

26. Buzard KA, Fundingsland BR. Excimer laser assisted in-situ keratomileusis for hyperopia. *J Cataract Ref Surg*. In press.

27. Kohenen T, Koch DD. Methods to control astigmatism in cataract surgery. *Curr Opin Ophthalmol*. 1996;7:75-80.

28. Samuelson SW, Koch DD, Kuglen CC. Determination of maximal incision length for true small-incision surgery. *Ophthalmic Surg*. 1991;22:204-7.

29. Personal communication with Maurice John.

30. Baikoff G, Colin J. IOLs in phakic patients. *Ophthalmol Clin North Am*. 1992;4:789-795.

31. Saragoussi JJ, Cotinat F, Renard M, et al. Damage to the corneal endothelium by minus power anterior chamber IOLs. *Refract Corneal Surg*. 1991;7:282-285.

32. Werblin TP. The long term endothelial cell loss following phacoemulsification surgery: The model for evaluating endothelial damage following intraocular surgery. *Refract Corneal Surg* 1993;9:29-35.

33. Clayman HM. IOLs. In Duane TD, ed: *Clinical Ophthalmology*. Vol 6. Philadelphia, Pa: Harper & Row; 1992;1-33.

34. Buzard KA, Fundingsland FB. Clear lens exchange for hyperopia. *Operative Techniques in Cataract and Refractive Surgery*. 1999;1:35-40.

35. Lyle WA, Jin CJC. Clear lens extraction for the correction of high refractive error. *J Cataract Refract Surg*. 1994;20:273-276.

36. Siganos SD, Siganos CS, Pallikaris IG. Clear lens extraction and IOL implantation in normally sighted hyperopic eyes. *J Refract Corneal Surg*. 1994;10:117-121.

37. Lindstrom RL. Retinal detachment in axial myopia. *Dev Ophthalmol*. 1987:14;37-41.

38. Praeger DL. Five years follow-up in the surgical management of cataracts in high myopia treated with the Kelman phacoemulsification technique. *Ophthalmology*. 1979;86:2024-2033.

39. Godberg MF. Clear lens extraction for axial myopia: An apprasial. *Ophthalmology*. 1987;94:571-5982.

40. Verzella F. Microsurgery of the lens in high myopia for optical purposes. *Cataract*. 1984;1:8-12.

41. Verzella F. High myopia: Refractive lensectomy and posterior chamber implants. *Cataract*. 1985;2:25-27.

42. Colin J, Robinet A. Clear lensectomy and implantation of low-power posterior chamber lens for the correction of high myopia. *Ophthalmology*. 1994;101:107-112.

43. Centurion V, Caballero JC, Medeiros OA, et al. Clear lens extraction and high myopia. In press.

44. Isfahani AH, Salz J. Clear lens extraction with IOL implantation for the correction of hyperopia. In: Shear ed *Surgery for Hyperopia and Presbyopia*. Baltimore, Md: Williams and Wilkins. 1997;175-181.

45. Siganos DS, Siganos CS, Pallikaris IG. Clear lens extraction and IOL implantation in normally sighted hyperopic eyes. *J Refract and Corneal Surg*. 1994;10:117-124.

46. Buzard KA. Clinical results of arcuate incisions to correct astigmatism. *J Cataract Refract Surg*. 1996;22:1062-69.

47. Buzard KA. Deepening of incisions after radial keratotomy using the "tickle technique." *J Refract and Corneal Surg*. 1991;5:348-55.

Index